Textbook of Dementia Care

T0231877

Textbook of Dementia Care: An Integrated Approach gives an overview of dementia care at a level appropriate to health and social care students, as well as providing an update to experienced practitioners. Authors come from a variety of backgrounds including nursing, psychiatry, medicine, psychology and allied health professions. There is a good mix of content from experienced new authors, academics and practitioners.

The book offers:

- a comprehensive list of contributors from different disciplines
- input from people living with dementia and their family carers
- relevant research to inform practice
- case examples to illustrate and inform the text.

While directed primarily at a nursing and social care readership, the book also provides a readable general text appropriate for all involved in dementia care. It is written by expert practitioners in the field, many of whom are leaders in practice-based research. It incorporates the expertise of representatives of Alzheimer Scotland but also includes accounts of people living with dementia, families, and carers, giving the reader a unique insight into the disease.

Graham A. Jackson is Emeritus Alzheimer Scotland Professor of Dementia Care at the University of the West of Scotland, UK.

Debbie Tolson is Alzheimer Scotland Professor of Dementia and Director of the Alzheimer Centre for Policy and Practice at the University of the West of Scotland, UK.

Textbook of Dementia Care

An Integrated Approach

Edited by
Graham A. Jackson and Debbie Tolson

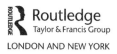

Routledge
Taylor & Francis Group

LONDON AND NEW YORK

First published 2019
by Routledge
2 Park Square, Milton Park, Abingdon, Oxon OX14 4RN

and by Routledge
52 Vanderbilt Avenue, New York, NY 10017

Routledge is an imprint of the Taylor & Francis Group, an informa business

British Library Cataloguing-in-Publication Data
A catalogue record for this book is available from the British Library

Library of Congress Cataloging-in-Publication Data
A catalog record has been requested for this book

ISBN: 978-1-138-22923-5 (hbk)
ISBN: 978-1-138-22924-2 (pbk)
ISBN: 978-1-315-38984-4 (ebk)

Typeset in Times New Roman
by Taylor & Francis Books

Printed and bound by CPI Group (UK) Ltd, Croydon, CR0 4YY

Contents

Figures

Tables

Foreword

This book makes a valuable contribution to the paradigm shift that continues to change and evolve our understanding of dementia. The text will help readers take dementia further out of the shadows; addressing the discrimination and stigma that still feature all too frequently in the lived experience of the illness. Alongside the political and policy developments that the authors highlight, the most important development in the past ten years has been the understanding that a person who happens to have a dementia diagnosis should, first and foremost, be recognised as an equal and valued citizen in their community. Irrespective of any drugs and other medical interventions that may be available, and no matter what non-pharmacological support we can offer, our driving principles must be the person with dementia's right to respect, dignity, choice, control and participation in our society.

Our global approach to dementia policy and practice has, for far too long, been dominated by the established, yet deeply problematic, medical model. This approach must change: here, now and with us. I am pleased to see that this text reflects the progressive, human rights-based movement that has been championed in Scotland; where policy, and increasingly practice, is driven by a fundamental belief in the rights to citizenship and inclusion.

The principles of human rights must underpin all skilled and thoughtful practice. We know that the provision of accurate, timely diagnosis, individualised post diagnostic support, effectively integrated community-based care and, ultimately, thoughtful and considered end-of-life and palliative care can, and will, be transformational for the person living with dementia and those closest to them. Is it too much to ask of our health and social care systems, of our society, that we not only recognise the value of this approach, but also commit to delivering it across Scotland and beyond?

The authors have given us a useful roadmap towards this vital goal. It is only by providing the best possible quality of care, support and practice as outlined in this text and underpinned by these principles that we can maintain this momentum and ensure the best possible quality of life for everyone living with dementia.

Henry Simmons
Chief Executive
Alzheimer Scotland

Contributors

Robert Boyd is a researcher and lecturer in Mental Health Nursing. He was formerly Dementia Nurse Consultant for NHS Tayside and maintains a research interest in the care of people with dementia, in particular in support for people newly diagnosed.

Dr Margaret Brown is Senior Lecturer and Depute Director of the Alzheimer Scotland Centre for Policy and Practice, University of the West of Scotland. Margaret is a researcher, educator and practitioner in the field of dementia, with a focus on education in advanced dementia. She has a lifetime achievement award for services to dementia care in Scotland.

Paul Brown is a Consultant liaison psychiatrist for older adults, NHS Greater Glasgow and Clyde, and Honorary Clinical Senior Lecturer, University of Glasgow, responsible for the psychiatric needs of older people in the general hospital and care homes. He has an interest in undergraduate education and in teaching organic psychiatry.

Arlene Crockett is Evidence and Influencing Co-ordinator, People Affected by Dementia Programme, The Life Changes Trust. Arlene joined the Life Changes trust in 2018 having worked for Alzheimer Scotland for the last 16 years, where she worked as a Service Manager and latterly as a Policy & Engagement Manager.

Adam Daly is a Consultant in Old Age Psychiatry, Chair of the Faculty of Old Age Psychiatry (Scotland) and Interim Associate Medical Director. Adam is an established consultant in Old Age Psychiatry working in Lanarkshire, Scotland. He has interests in service development and improvement related to mental health, and older adults.

F. J. Raymond Duffy is Programme leader for the MSc in Gerontology and MSc in Gerontology (with Dementia Care) at the University of the West of Scotland. He has been an educator and practitioner in older people's care throughout his career. His main interest is the impact of long-term illnesses, including dementia, on the lives of older people.

Graham Ellis is a Consultant Geriatrician, NHS Lanarkshire and Honorary Professor, Glasgow Caledonian University School of Life and Health Sciences. He is a Geriatrician in NHS Lanarkshire in Central Scotland and a clinician with a research interest in the organisation of acute services for older people.

Irene Graham is an Administration Manager for Mental Health currently working with NHS Ayrshire and Arran. She was a carer for her husband for over 12 years.

Rekha Hegde is a Consultant Old Age Psychiatrist Clinical lead Old Age Liaison service NHS Lanarkshire. Dr Hegde has looked after older people's mental health for the last 11 years. She is a Regional advisor, and is on the Specialty Advisory Committee for Old Age Psychiatry.

Jenny Henderson is an Associate Lecturer University of the West of Scotland. Jenny has over 30 years' experience of working with people with dementia both in health and social care her specific area of interest is advanced dementia. In 2018 she was awarded the UWS Celebration medal.

Guy Holloway is a Consultant in Old Age Psychiatry, Royal Edinburgh Hospital. Dr Holloway trained as a GP and then in Psychiatry. He has worked as a Consultant in Old Age Psychiatry since 2002 and has a particular interest in reducing inappropriate prescribing.

Graham A. Jackson is Emeritus Professor at the Alzheimer Scotland Centre for Policy and Practice, part of the School of Health and Life Sciences at the University of the West of Scotland. Graham is interested in research in the field of dementia, particularly service delivery. Before joining UWS he was a consultant in Old Age Psychiatry in NHS Greater Glasgow and Clyde.

Amanda Johnson is a Clinical Nurse Manager, NHS Ayrshire & Arran. Amanda is an RGN and has worked in various roles and clinical settings within NHS Ayrshire & Arran. She was Dementia Improvement Lead with the Scottish Focus on Dementia programme for two years.

Lindsay Kinnaird is Research Manager, Alzheimer Scotland. Lindsay has collaborated on and led the development of a number of public policy publications. These have covered the different phases of dementia and included community settings and specialist hospital care.

Stephen Lithgow is an Occupational Therapist with Greater Glasgow and Clyde NHS. He has worked as a Dementia Support and Development Lead in Glasgow in dementia research, strategy, and Post Diagnosis Support. He is presently on secondment as an Associate Improvement Advisor with the Focus on Dementia Team at Healthcare Improvement Scotland working with Specialist Dementia Units.

Donald Lyons is a retired Consultant Psychiatrist and former Chief Executive of the Mental Welfare Commission for Scotland. He has published extensively on ethical care of people with dementia and other mental health conditions. He received a lifetime achievement award at the Scottish Dementia Awards 2014.

Ajay Verma Macharouthu is Consultant in Liaison Psychiatry for the Elderly, NHS Ayrshire & Arran and Honorary Clinical Senior Lecturer, University of Glasgow. He is Scottish Delirium Association Chair and co-chairs the SIGN Delirium group. Interests include interprofessional teaching and dementia research.

Mary Marshall is Honorary Professor at the University of Edinburgh and emeritus at the University of Stirling. She is a senior consultant with the Dementia Centre Hammond Care, specialising in enabling design for people with dementia.

Trudi Marshall is Associate Director of Nursing Health and Social Care Partnership North Lanarkshire. She is a registered nurse with over 25 years' experience. She has worked in a variety of older peoples' services and has a passion for ensuring services meet the needs of older people.

Janice McAlister is a Dementia Nurse Consultant currently working at Erskine. She trained as an RMN at NHS Ayrshire & Arran. Receiving a BSc Hons in Community Nursing from UWS and MSc in Dementia from Stirling University.

James McKillop was a founding member of the Scottish Dementia Working Group, a campaigning group of people with dementia that is supported by Alzheimer Scotland. He was awarded the MBE in 2011, and an Honorary Doctorate from the University of Strathclyde in 2013 for services to people with dementia.

Bryan Mitchell is a Lecturer in the School of Health and Life Sciences. Bryan's background and research interest are in complementary healthcare where he has experience of working in long-term care facilities for individual with later stage dementia using tailored interventions.

Mike Nolan is Honorary Chair in Gerontological Nursing at the University of Sheffield. For the past 30 years he has explored ways of improving services for older people, family carers and staff using a relationship-centred approach.

Sam Quinn is a social researcher at the University of the West of Scotland. His research interests include learning disability, dementia and palliative care.

Louise Ritchie is a Lecturer in Dementia (Research), Alzheimer Scotland Centre for Policy and Practice, University of the West of Scotland. Louise is a lecturer with a focus on applied dementia research. Louise's academic background is in psychology and her current work focuses on dementia and employment, and psychosocial interventions in dementia care.

Tony Ryan is Reader in Older People, Care and the Family at the University of Sheffield. He has been carrying out research in the field of health and social care for and with people with dementia for the past 20 years. Focusing on relationships and day-to-day experiences he has an interest in community-based support and palliative care for families affected by dementia.

Sandra Shafii is a Consultant in the Technology Enabled Care & Digital Healthcare Innovation Division. Sandra is a state registered occupational therapist. She has held a range of clinical and managerial roles including General Manager, Lead Clinician and National Allied Health Professions Dementia Consultant.

Dr Barbara Sharp is Nurse Lecturer, Practice Educator, Policy and Practice Consultant with Alzheimer Scotland. Barbara supports the rights and care of people with dementia across Scotland through education, research, partnership working, policy development and application.

Henry Simmons is Chief Executive, Alzheimer Scotland.

Christine Steel is an Allied Health Professional Dementia Consultant. After a successful appointment to a seconded Scottish Government funded post as National AHP Dementia Consultant, Christine is now the AHP Dementia Consultant for NHS Greater Glasgow & Clyde.

Lucy Stirland is a Clinical Research Fellow in Old Age Psychiatry. Lucy is a Specialty Registrar in Old Age Psychiatry and Clinical Research Fellow at the University of Edinburgh, where she investigates interactions between physical and mental health in ageing

Debbie Tolson is Alzheimer Scotland Professor of Dementia and Director of the Alzheimer Centre for Policy and Practice at the University of the West of Scotland. The focus of Debbie's nursing career has been the promotion of evidence informed practice that enables individuals and families to live the best life possible.

Karen Watchman is a Senior Lecturer, Faculty of Health Sciences and Sport, University of Stirling. Karen has worked with people who have a learning disability and their families for many years in both practice and academic settings. She teaches and provides training on learning disability and dementia in the UK and internationally.

Anna Jack-Waugh is a Lecturer in Dementia Alzheimer Scotland Centre for Policy and Practice. Anna has extensive experience care of people living with dementia and education of staff. She also teaches into the undergraduate and postgraduate nursing programmes and leads Scotland's National Dementia Champions programme team.

Part I
Dementia in context

1 Introduction

Graham A. Jackson and Debbie Tolson

In the last decade public and political interest in dementia and dementia care has increased greatly. Calls for research to prevent, treat and cure dementia abound, and governments around the world have been charged with creating national dementia action plans (European Parliament 2010) and to invest in the development of the dementia workforce and to improve services (Department of Health 2013). The World Health Organisation Global Dementia Action Plan 2017 is for people with dementia and their carers to live well and receive the care and support they need to fulfil their potential to live with dignity, respect, autonomy and equality (World Health Organisation 2017). This improvement imperative is particularly welcomed by individuals, family and practitioners, many of whom have direct experience of what might be described as the inverse care law, that is to say, that those who need most care seem to receive least (Tolson et al. 2016).

To address such inequalities and to accelerate evidence informed person-centred care will require a commitment to both integrated expert led practice and integrated specialist services. This repositioning of dementia care as specialist and complex is a prerequisite for progress that calls for a greater and more nuanced understanding of the underlying cause, illness trajectory and its impact on the person's life.

What is dementia? The definition from the World Health Organisation (Box 1.1) is widely used. As we can see it is not one condition, but a syndrome that can be caused by a number of different diseases all of which cause significant brain damage. The commonest form is Alzheimer's disease; other common forms are vascular dementia, Lewy Body dementia and frontotemporal dementia. Other forms are much less common. We know that dementia incidence increases with age, so, as the average age of population rises, so too will the number of people with dementia.

Box 1.1 Learning point: Definition of dementia

Dementia is a syndrome due to disease of the brain, usually of a chronic or progressive nature, in which there is disturbance of multiple higher cortical functions, including memory, thinking, orientation, comprehension, calculation, learning capacity, language, and judgement. Consciousness is not clouded. The impairments of cognitive function are commonly accompanied, and occasionally preceded, by deterioration in emotional control, social behaviour, or motivation. This syndrome occurs in Alzheimer disease, in cerebrovascular disease, and in other conditions primarily or secondarily affecting the brain.

(World Health Organisation, 1999)

However, these conditions are often not easy to separate from one another. There is a lot of overlap in how they present and indeed even brain imaging is still not accurate. At the present state of medical knowledge, it is perhaps less important to put a definitive label on the type of dementia, as there are no specific and effective treatments. Although diagnosis will help determination and anticipation of patterns of need and inform advances in more specific tailoring of caring and treatment interventions. A diagnosis of Lewy body dementia, for example, is important when prescribing medication due to potential responses to drugs both in terms of side effects and in terms of targeting specific symptoms that can be very important. For people who develop dementia earlier in life there are strong genetic factors at work, so it is important to know the nature of the dementia for planning their care and in providing their offspring with information about their own dementia risks and life choices.

Although we generally think of dementia as a condition of later life, and age is indeed a risk factor, it may start earlier in life. Various phrases are used from time to time to describe the rise in the number of people with dementia, such as the dementia epidemic, the rising tide, the ticking time bomb. But the use of these terms contributes to the stigma dementia has in society. More people with dementia in society is the result of a success story, of people living longer and remaining generally healthier. We must also remember that particularly in Western societies much of the reported rise can be explained by better and more efficient diagnostic pathways.

Writing now in 2018, no drugs have been licensed for the treatment of dementia since the late 1990s. There are a lot of potential compounds being investigated, but not available for general use. Many promising avenues of research have proved fruitless. One of the difficulties though is that we do not really understand the brain mechanisms of normal functioning, let alone why they go wrong. Failure of many promising avenues, including preventative studies, are hampered by the fact that the disease process in the brain is likely to have started several decades before the onset of symptoms.

It has been increasingly recognised that Alzheimer's disease and vascular dementia share common risk factors with cardiovascular conditions in general including smoking, poor diet, high blood pressure, lack of exercise and family history. Changes in the incidence from stroke disease and heart attacks in Western countries are being followed by a potential drop in the expected numbers of people with dementia, emphasising the role of preventative factors.

So, in the future we may see treatments which prevent or at least ameliorate the effects of dementia. This is likely though to be a long way off, if indeed it does happen. However, the current challenge for society is one of making sure that people with dementia are able to live the best life possible throughout the various stages of illness from onset to the end of their lives.

The definition of dementia referred to above focuses on impairments, on what people are unable to do. While it is important to recognise that there is neurological damage which does affect how someone is able to manage in life, at the same time we should look to build on individual capabilities. A person's abilities and needs will change across the continuum of their life with dementia. Dementia does not exempt a person from other health problems and illnesses, and these must be taken into account within dementia care planning, and managed appropriately. Dementia is a progressive condition that most commonly affects memory, cognition, communication and sensory experiences. It gives rise to complex physical health needs, psychosocial needs and spiritual and existential needs. Accordingly, it follows that integrated models of care, that recognise and responds to these range of evolving needs, both of the individual, and of their family, is likely to yield better outcomes than non-integrated alternatives.

As a society we must ensure that people are not stigmatised by having dementia, and recognise that people have a right to the most rewarding and fulfilling life possible by providing appropriate integrated care and support to them and their families whenever and wherever it is needed. This will only be possible with commitment, creativity and involvement of everyone from politicians, to planners, to practitioners and researchers, to designers, to people who provide care, to families and of course to people with dementia themselves.

This book is intended to help people to fulfil this aim.

References

Department of Health (2013) "G8 dementia summit agreements." Available from: https://www.gov.uk/government/publications/g8-dementia-summit-agreements.

European Parliament (2010) "Report on a European initiative on Alzheimer's disease and other dementias (2010/2084(INI))." Available from: http://www.europarl.europa.eu/sides/getDoc.do?pubRef=-//EP//NONSGML+REPORT+A7-2010-0366+0+DOC+PDF+V0//EN.

Tolson, D., Flemming, A., Hanson, E., de Abreu, W., Lillo Crespo, M., MacRae, R., Jackson, G.A., Touzery, S.H., Routasalo, P., Holmerová, I. (2016). "Achieving Prudent Dementia Care (Palliare): an international policy and practice imperative." *International Journal of Integrated Care*. doi:10.5334/ijic.2497.

World Health Organisation (1999) "The International Statistical Classification of Diseases and Related Health Problems (ICD 10)." Available from: https://icd.who.int/browse10/2016/en.

World Health Organisation (2017) "WHO Global Dementia Plan." Available from: http://apps.who.int/gb/ebwha/pdf_files/EB140/B140_28-en.pdf?ua=1.

Further reading

Ritchie, C.W., Russ, T.C., Banerjee, S., Barber, B., Boaden, A., Fox, N.C., Holmes, C., Isaacs, J. D., Leroi, I., Lovestone, S., Norton, M., O'Brien, J., Pearson, J., Perry, R., Pickett, J., Waldman, A.D., Wong, W.L., Rossor, M.N., Burns, A. *(*2017) "The Edinburgh Consensus: preparing for the advent of disease-modifying therapies for Alzheimer's disease." *Alzheimer's Research & Therapy* 9(85). Available from: https://doi.org/10.1186/s13195-017-0312-4.

2   Policy perspectives

Graham A. Jackson, Debbie Tolson and Lindsay Kinnaird

Dementia has gradually over the past two decades or so been recognised as a major issue globally (Prince et al. 2013). Developments in health and social care as well as a rise in wealth across the world have led to an increase in the average lifespan. While this is most evident in the so-called western world, this is happening in most if not all countries. Particularly rapid increases in the numbers and proportion of older people are forecast for China, India, and Latin America (Sousa et al. 2010). The main risk factor for the development of dementia is of course advancing age, so an older population means many more people living with dementia.

The increasing numbers of people living with dementia combined with the economic challenges which many countries have been facing have led to predictions that care and treatment will become unaffordable if they continue to be developed and provided using current models. International developments to try to address this have included the G8 Dementia Summit in 2013, chaired by the then British Prime Minister David Cameron, and the 2015 World Health Organisation (WHO) Ministerial Conference on Global Action Against Dementia.

In 2015 Alzheimer's Disease International released their annual World Alzheimer Report focussing on the global effects of dementia and provided estimates of the prevalence and consequences of dementia up until 2050. It suggested that almost 50 million people were living with dementia in 2015 and predicted that this would treble by 2050, with by far the biggest rises in low- and middle- income countries. While many recent studies have suggested that the rate of increase in dementia is slowing, there is no doubt that providing support will continue to be a major challenge, and absolute numbers will continue to increase significantly by virtue of the increasing older population.

Changes in the make-up of society also put an increased burden on state and self-provided support. Social mobility has led to a great decrease in what has been referred to as familial piety, that is, the dealing of problems of health and social support within one's own networks and families. Extended families are less likely to stay near to the family home than was the case only a few decades ago, and families are increasingly fractured with the traditional model of support less likely to be available.

In the UK, the expectations we have of receiving good quality care throughout our lives has grown. No longer is the Shakespearean description of old age (from *As You Like It*) "Last scene of all… is second childishness and mere oblivion, sans teeth, sans eyes, sans taste, sans everything" seen as reality for ourselves. Yet we still talk in terms of the elderly as being a different group from ourselves, rather than as us when we grow older. This is partly why politicians throughout the world do not plan in terms of how to fund support. They are reactive, tending to look at the here and now only. It is difficult to feel confident of being reelected if politicians tell people that their taxes will have to rise, or that other services will have to be cut, to fund care for "the elderly". Yet that is what is going to have to happen.

In many health services, a good example being the UK, there is a principal that health care will be free at the point of need. While this works reasonably well when it is for emergency or short-term care, it is increasingly difficult to provide in the long term. In Scotland the government introduced free personal care for people over the age of 65 in the early part of the 21st century. This means that some aspects of personal care are funded, for all who need it, by the state. It can be argued though that this particularly benefits those with their own resources, as the state has always funded such support for those who were totally unable to afford it. Whatever the rights and wrongs, increasing numbers of people being entitled to it, and therefore the cost, means that this policy is increasingly under scrutiny.

In many countries there are insurance-based schemes to help provide care. But these too are expensive, and lead to a two-tier system of care where those on low income rely on what is often second-rate care, while those who are well insured may be subjected to expensive and perhaps not strictly necessary investigations and treatment. Systems to pay for long-term care are often different from those with acute care. In the USA for example most of the population insure for medical expenses in general, but only a small number have policies covering long-term care.

Many countries in Europe and to a lesser extent across the rest of the world have a National Dementia Plan of some kind. This is often termed a National Dementia Strategy. The purpose of these plans is to drive improvements of the support for people with dementia at all stages of their illness. They tend to follow similar themes and have generally been developed by governments with involvement of people with dementia, their carers and professionals who work with them. In Scotland, the strategy was developed after the production of a charter of rights for people with dementia: many other countries have followed this lead. Dementia strategies are relatively recent additions to policy, and moving from strategy to local implementation still needs a lot of work. In 2014 at a conference in Glasgow Alzheimer Europe published the Glasgow declaration (see Box 2.3), calling for world leaders to recognise dementia as a public health priority and to develop a global action plan on dementia (see Box 2.1).

Box 2.1 Learning point: Dementia Plans

Dementia Plans generally call for increased recognition of dementia at an early stage, with prompt and efficient diagnostic pathways and support for the person with dementia and their families and carers to live the best life possible. There seems little doubt that it is a good thing to do, to diagnose dementia as early in its trajectory as possible; yet in the absence of effective treatments, the benefits of this are largely in terms of enabling the person with dementia and those around them to access support when necessary, and to make plans for the future. This includes making plans for who will make decisions on their behalf once the person with dementia is unable to by making someone a proxy, such as a Power of Attorney. The evidence for this making a difference in terms of outcomes though is at present limited.

For people with established dementia there is an increased emphasis on living well in the community. This includes making communities more dementia-friendly, as well as enabling people with dementia to participate in their previous activities and indeed to develop new ones. In England and to a lesser extent Scotland the Dementia Friends programme has helped make many more people dementia aware. There is also a general recognition that the care of people with dementia in general hospitals is far from ideal, a hospital is not the best place for a person with dementia to be. Initiatives here include Scotland's Dementia Champions Programme that is increasing the skills in dealing with dementia of non-specialist nurses and others.

Box 2.2 Learning point: Stigma

Tackling the stigma associated with dementia is key to how the illness is viewed within society. Equally recognising the rights of the person with dementia is important in providing good quality care and treatment. Initiatives such as dementia-friendly communities demonstrate that raising public awareness and understanding of the illness can promote everyday approaches in supporting people participate in society. The responses of others are of key importance in honouring the continued recognition of personhood and the needs of the person with dementia.

The challenges of dealing with the rising number of older people, and dementia generally, have led to increasing calls for what has been termed prudent healthcare, that is, the rational use of evidence-based practice with healthcare which fits with the patients' needs and avoiding unnecessary health inputs (Tolson et al. 2016).

Many people with dementia spend the last days of their lives in nursing homes, or in their own homes with limited professional support. While the hospice movement has made great strides internationally in improving support and care for those in the terminal stages of cancer, such support for those with dementia lags behind. Caring for older people is often seen as a low status occupation, with subsequent poor rates of pay, poor training opportunities and poor career progression, all leading potentially to poor morale.

In recent years there has been an increased focus on prevention of dementia, and further work on the development of treatments. Evidence for this having made much difference at present however is largely lacking. The possible availability of effective drugs will mean the development of more effective pathways for pre-clinical diagnosis. This is described in the Edinburgh Consensus (Ritchie et al. 2017), though how this would be funded is not addressed.

Advanced dementia presents a range of complex health issues in addition to the social and psychological impact of the illness. Health care practitioners have a key role in responding to the increasing physical nature of the illness. Equally palliative care has an important supporting role in the advanced phase of illness and at end of life. However, people with dementia do not gain access to the range of multi-professionals required to address the complexity of the illness.

Concerted government action is required at a national and local level in order to develop appropriate support. Dementia is complex with health and social care needs intensifying as the illness progresses. The increased emphasis on supporting people to live well in the community requires a coordinated approach that responds to the needs of the individual. However, too often support is fragmented and fails to address the full range of needs in a structured way.

Box 2.3 Learning point: Glasgow Declaration

As signatories, we commit ourselves fully to promoting the rights, dignity and *autonomy* of people living with dementia. These rights are universal, and guaranteed in the European Convention of Human Rights, the Universal Declaration of Human Rights, the International Covenants on Economic, Social and Cultural Rights and Civil and Political Rights, and the Convention on the Rights of Persons with Disabilities.

We affirm that every person living with dementia has:

- The right to a timely *diagnosis*;
- The right to access quality post diagnostic support;
- The right to person-centred, coordinated, quality care throughout their illness;
- The right to equitable access to treatments and therapeutic interventions;
- The right to be respected as an individual in their community.

We welcome the growing recognition of dementia as a public health priority on a national and European level and call upon European governments and institutions to recognise the role that they have in ensuring that these rights of people living with dementia are respected and upheld. In particular, we:

- Call upon the European Commission to:

1   Develop a European Dementia Strategy;
2   Designate a high level EU official to coordinate the activities and research in the field of dementia of existing programmes such as Horizon 2020, the Ambient Assisted Living Programme, the European Innovation Partnership on Active and Healthy Ageing, the Joint Programme on Neurodegenerative diseases research and the Innovative Medicines Initiative;
3   Set up a European Expert Group on Dementia comprised of Commission officials, representatives of Member States and civil society to exchange best practices;
4   Financially support the activities of Alzheimer Europe and its European Dementia Observatory and European Dementia Ethics Network through its public health programme.

- Call upon Members of the European Parliament to:

1   Join the European Alzheimer's Alliance;
2   Support the campaign of Alzheimer Europe and its member organisations to make dementia a European priority and create a European Dementia Strategy;
3   Make themselves available for people with dementia, carers and representatives of Alzheimer associations from their country.

- Call upon national governments to:

1   Develop comprehensive national dementia strategies with allocated funding and a clear monitoring and evaluation process;
2   Involve people living with dementia and their carers in the development and follow up of these national strategies;
3   Support national Alzheimer and dementia associations.

We welcome the international recognition of dementia as global priority and acknowledge the work of Alzheimer's Disease International and the G7 group of countries in driving forward global action on dementia and call upon the international community to:

1   Build on the success of European collaboration on dementia and involve European initiatives in the development of a global action plan on dementia;
2   Include and consult Alzheimer associations and people with dementia in the decision making process and definition of a global research agenda;
3   Adopt a holistic approach to research priorities to include psycho-social, care, socio-economic and health systems research to ensure that research aims to benefit people living with dementia now, as well as people who will do so in years to come;
4   Substantially increase the funding dedicated to all areas of dementia research;
5   Promote dementia as a priority in other international bodies including among the G20 group of countries, the Organisation for Economic Co-operation and Development (OECD), the World Health Organisation (WHO) and the United Nations.

(Alzheimer Europe 2014)

References

Alzheimer Europe (2014) "The Glasgow declaration." Available from: www.alzheimer-europe. org/Policy-in-Practice2/Glasgow-Declaration-2014.

Prince, M., Bryce, R., Albanese, E., Wimo, A., Ribeiro, W., Ferri, C.P. (2013) "The global prevalence of dementia: A systematic review and metanalysis." *Alzheimer's & Dementia* 9(1): 63–75. http://doi.org/10.1016/j.jalz.2012.11.007.

Ritchie, C.W., Russ, T.C., Banerjee, S., Barber, B., Boaden, A., Fox, N.C., Holmes, C., Isaacs, J. D., Leroi, I., Lovestone, S., Norton, M., O'Brien, J., Pearson, J., Perry, R., Pickett, J., Waldman, A.D., Wong, W.L., Rossor, M.N., Burns, A. (2017) "The Edinburgh Consensus: preparing for the advent of disease-modifying therapies for Alzheimer's disease." *Alzheimer's Research & Therapy* 9(85). Available from: https://doi.org/10.1186/s13195-017-0312-4.

Sousa, R.M., Ferri, C.P., Acosta, M.G., Guerra, M., Huang, Y., Jacob, K.S., Jotheeswaran, A. T., Guerra Hernandez, M.A., Liuz Pichardo, G.R., Rodriguez, J.J.L., Salas, A., Sosa, A.L., Williams, J., Zuniga, T., Prince, M. (2010) "The contribution of chronic diseases to the prevalence of dependence among older people in Latin America, China and India: A 10/66 Dementia Research Group population-based survey." *BMC Geriatr* 10(53). doi:10.1186/1471-2318-10-doi:53.

Tolson, D., Flemming, A., Hanson, E., de Abreu, W., Lillo Crespo, M., MacRae, R., Jackson, G.A., Touzery, S.H., Routasalo, P., Holmerová, I. (2016). "Achieving Prudent Dementia Care (Palliare): an international policy and practice imperative." *International Journal of Integrated Care.* doi:10.5334/ijic.2497.

Further reading

Alzheimer Europe (2017) "Comparing and benchmarking national dementia strategies and policies." *European Dementia Monitor 2017*. Available from: https://www.alzheimer-europe.org/ Publications/E-Shop/European-Dementia-Monitor-2017/European-Dementia-Monitor-2017.

3   Relationships, values and dementia care

Promoting reciprocity and interdependence

Tony Ryan and Mike Nolan

> If employees are abandoned and abused, probably clients will be too. If employees are supported and encouraged they will take their sense of well-being into their day-to-day work.
>
> (Kitwood 1997)

Introduction

The above sentiments are as relevant today as they were almost 20 years ago. The intervening period has seen multiple public investigations into the quality of care vulnerable people receive that have shaken the health and social care landscape to the core. Many of these enquiries have focussed on services for older people and specifically those living with dementia and their families. Standards of care for these groups are still regularly called into question despite the policy and practice rhetoric espousing the person-centred values that Tom Kitwood (1997) promoted some two decades ago. Mission statements and organisational values are now routinely framed using a person-centred discourse that permeates services and consequently health and social care providers all aspire to deliver care that maintains and enables personhood. However, this is manifestly not being achieved and by exploring the relationship between values and care in a dementia context this chapter considers why such practice continues to exist. We argue that values are pivotal to the ways in which care is conceptualised and delivered. A relationship-centred model recognises the importance of creating "enriched" environments for people with dementia, family carers and staff. This model is underpinned by the "senses framework" (Nolan et al. 2006) and suggests that it is timely for us to reconsider the boundaries of such thinking to move beyond care settings and into the physical and social life of communities. The current rhetoric of "care" and the values of independence and autonomy inadvertently place people with dementia in a dependent position and we need to create environments in which the contribution of the person is recognised and sustained for as long as possible. This will mean a shift from values such as independence and autonomy towards interdependence, reciprocity and the centrality of the notion of the contribution that people with dementia can make to our organisations and communities. We begin by briefly examining the notion of person-centred care, recognising, as have others, the seminal contribution made by Kitwood (Baldwin et al. 2007), and subsequently outline the emergence of relationship centred care and the "senses framework", considering the implications of the latter for the development of environments that can maximise the contribution of people with dementia, family carers and staff who support them.

Person-centred care

According to Adams and Bartlett (2003) two discourses dominated the ways in which dementia was conceptualised in the 20th century, the bio-medical and the cognitive models. The former focussed on the identification and classification of neurophysiological and neurochemical changes in the brains of people with dementia, the latter on how dementia impacts on cognitive functioning and specifically memory performance.

However both discourses were challenged by the notion of person-centred dementia care advanced by the late Tom Kitwood (1997) who argued for a new approach to understanding dementia that was concerned with the:

> dialectical interplay between neurological impairment and malignant social psychology.
>
> (Adams and Bartlett 2003, 98)

At the core of Kitwood's model lies the belief that the personhood of the person with dementia remains present throughout and is a product of the interactions between: their physical health, their biography, their network of their social relationships and their neurological impairment. For Kitwood (1997) assisting people with dementia to find meaning in their illness contributes to the preservation of their personhood and aim should underpin good care.

It is true to say that Kitwood's work has transformed dementia care over the last two decades by placing the *person* with dementia at the centre and reaffirming their worth and intrinsic value as an individual. More recently however Hughes (2013) has identified a further "philosophical" shift in how the experience of dementia is portrayed, one in which relationships are now seen as pivotal. This marks, as Morhardt and Spira (2013) note, a gradual move over time away from a person-centred model towards a more inclusive relationship-centred approach. Whilst the focus of this latter model was initially on dyadic relationships, primarily between spousal couples (Hellström et al. 2007; Molyneaux et al. 2012; Balfour 2014) attention has since expanded to include the wider family (Roach et al. 2012) and beyond (Toms et al. 2015). These developments are of more than theoretical interest and have resulted in calls for "relationship work" to be a recognised from of intervention for couples and others living with dementia (Molyneaux et al. 2012; Balfour 2014).

Despite this shift in the way that dementia is thought about by some commentators, changes have yet to fully inform either policy or practice. This is apparent in the ways in which recent major policy initiatives such as "Dementia-Friendly Communities" (Department of Health 2015) and the Dementia Action Alliance (2014) continue to adopt an almost exclusively individualistic discourse with the focus remaining firmly on the person with dementia. This is captured below by how the Dementia Action Alliance, an England wide network of people and organisations committed to improving health and social care provision for people affected by dementia, which argues for a "society wide response." They see this as being achieved when a person with dementia can say:

- I have personal choice and control or influence over decisions about me
- I know that services are designed around me and my needs
- I have support that helps me live my life
- I have the knowledge and know-how to get what I need
- I have a sense of belonging and of being a valued part of family, community and civic life
- I live in an enabling and supportive environment where I feel valued and understood
- I know there is research going on which delivers a better life for me now and hope for the future.

(Dementia Action Alliance 2014)

Whilst these aims appear highly laudable and it seems counter-intuitive to argue against them it is the overwhelming emphasis on "I" and "me" that, for us, represents the Achilles heel at the centre of person-centred models.

Whilst fully recognising the seminal contribution made by Kitwood, even his former collaborators have begun to argue for an extended vision of personhood and have questioned the place it accords people with dementia. The editors of a volume celebrating, but also turning a critical gaze on Kitwoods work, suggest that his vision of personhood was rather unidirectional in that it saw personhood as something conferred on people with dementia **by others** without explicitly acknowledging the ways in which people with dementia may themselves confer personhood. They sum this up as follows:

Although the proposed theory of personhood is relational, Kitwood only captures a unidirectional realization of that theory. Consequently, the theory and its realization in person-centred care are individualistic and focussed on the person living with dementia to the exclusion of those caring for that person living with dementia. Thus the theory is uneven in the sense that people living with dementia have personhood bestowed on them but are not seen as bestowing personhood on others. They are thus made more dependent on and vulnerable to the vicissitudes of others.

(Baldwin et al. 2007, 181)

These authors go on to argue whilst Kitwood stressed that people with dementia "matter" he did not adequately explore their potential to be active agents in their own right, nor did he fully consider how the experiences of people with dementia may be shaped by the socio-political context, nor how they might be able to influence that context themselves (Baldwin et al. 2007).

Recently several authors have proposed a wider approach which accords people with dementia a more active and more integrated role, stressing the fact that rather than being largely passive recipients care that people with dementia can and do make an active contribution, reciprocating in multiple ways. For example Dupuis et al. (2011) stress that "synergisitic relationships" based on interdependence and reciprocity are essential to the creation of "authentic partnerships" between people with dementia, families and service systems. Simlarly van Gennip et al. (2014) argue that if people with dementia are to maintain their dignity and identity then attention must be turned to three domains. They describe these in the following ways:

- The "inter-personal dimension" in which it is vital to create an environment in which people with dementia can still engage in meaningful activity
- The "relational-self" and the importance of facilitating interactions in which, although perhaps increasingly dependent on others, people with dementia are still able to reciprocate
- The "social-self", comprising interactions with the outside world. This is seen as the most challenging arena, and the one in which a negative experience has the greatest potential to reduced dignity.

The above reflect concepts such "social worth" in which people with dementia remain active contributors at multiple levels, with Robertson (2014) stressing that in order to do so people with dementia need to both build on prior relationships and also develop new ones:

> Finding meaning (when living with dementia) therefore depends on maintaining connections with valued roles and relationships from the past and establishing roles and relationships that bring a new sense of purpose to life.
>
> (Robertson 2014, 538)

Ideas such as those promoted above, that were developed specifically with people with dementia in mind, mirror other recent work that has focussed on what creates a meaningful life for older people with "high support needs" (Katz et al. 2011). Building on a raft of studies conducted over many years the Joseph Rowntree Foundation have identified seven key challenges to improving the well-being and contribution of people with high support needs (Blood 2013). The importance of relationships figures prominently as a key challenge, as captured by Blood below:

> We must ensure that all support is founded in, and reflects, meaningful relationships. Connecting with others is a fundamental human need, whatever our age or support needs.
>
> (Blood 2013, 13)

The work of Katz et al. (2011) and others (e.g. Tanner 2010) credits older people, including those with high support needs, with having agency and of being able to actively "manage" their lives. Key concepts, such as resilience in older age are now emerging (Wiles et al. 2011) that again highlight the vital role played by social relationships and connections with community, rather than physical/ mental functioning or socio-economic status, in capturing the interactional and contextual nature of ageing.

Although recent conceptualisations of person-centred care have taken a more inclusive approach (see for example McCormack and McCance 2010; Brooker and Latham 2016) they still do not, for us, explicitly acknowledge the value and importance of interdependence, integration and reciprocity that lie at the heart of a relationship centred approach. It is such a model that we promote here and is particularly important given the care integration agenda.

From person to relationship centred care

Most modern day societies, especially in the developed, Western world, are underpinned by the core values of independence and autonomy. As a consequence key goals of their health, and to a lesser extent social, care systems revolve around enabling people to maintain function and fulfil "productive" social roles. Such aspirations are by the promotion of concepts such as "successful" ageing (Rowe and Kahn 1997) and the World Health Organisation's global policy of achieving "Active Ageing" (WHO 2002). Gerontologists have long argued that such goals disadvantage older people who cannot meet the criteria for success (usually associated with high levels of physical and mental functioning and the absence of disease (Clarke and Warren 2007)). This would certainly be true of people with dementia.

The need for an alternative model of care provision, particularly one that can meet with the challenges posed by the rise in long-term conditions, was recognised some two decades ago by a major task force considering the future of health care in the USA (Tresolini and Pew-Fetzer Task Force 1994). They concluded that any effective system for the future must be based on a relationship-centred model that explicitly acknowledges that "the interactions amongst people (are) the foundation of any therapeutic or healing activity. The concept of relationship centred care (RCC) emerged as a consequence. However, whilst the taskforce provided a broad conceptual vision of what RCC might look like, they did not, as they acknowledge, propose a means by which such a model might be realised in practice.

To fill this gap extensive work conducted over a 15-year period resulted in the initial development, refinement and application of a framework for RCC, the "Senses Framework" (Nolan et al. 2006). At the heart of this framework lies the goal of creating an "enriched environment". Such an environment is one in which **all** those involved, for example people with dementia, family members and paid staff experience six "senses" (Nolan et al. 2006).

These six senses are:

A sense of security – to feel safe and secure, not just physically but also psychologically.
A sense of belonging – to feel "part of things", to be able to maintain existing relationships and to form new ones.
A sense of continuity – to know that your biography and life history are recognised and valued
A sense of purpose – having valued goals to aim for and to feel that "I have a contribution to make."
A sense of achievement – being enabled to achieve valued goals and to feel satisfied, and recognised for, with your efforts.
A sense of significance – to feel that you "matter" and your existence counts for something.

Figure 3.1 The senses framework

Since this framework was originally proposed it has been applied to a wide range of settings and with numerous groups, including people with dementia, their families and staff (Ryan et al. 2008).

Whilst the "senses" framework has been widely adopted over recent years it has been primarily underpinned by the concept of care. Whilst highly relevant in certain situations in others this places some parties in an implicitly dependent position. This may to a degree be inevitable when high levels of support are needed if people with dementia are to play as full a role as possible, for as long as possible we would suggest that the notion of an enriched environment should be extended to consider how the creation of the "senses" can enable all parties to make their maximum **contribution.** It is this that we now go on to consider for people with dementia, families and staff.

There is a well-established literature recognising the reciprocal nature of caregiving situations. Indeed it is argued that caregiving relationships can only be sustained where there exists an exchange of reward and satisfaction. Marck (1990) considers the nature of the therapeutic relationship via the notion of mutuality in a range of forms, from the recognition of the exchange of humour through to the disclosure of personal information, arguing that these human processes are essential to the formation of trust and empathy. Furthermore, Marck's ideas at the time helped to transform thinking about care from a linear "passive" experience to one where both parties achieve a "mutual exchange" where the "costs of care" are transformed into "positive growth" for the caregiver and cared for person (Marck 1990, 51). Such transformative thinking allows for a recognition of the role of people with dementia in care encounters, albeit often hidden and under-explored. Our own work identified these experiences for care workers in that their motivations and satisfactions derived from the work was based upon shared experiences and viewed as a "joint venture". The contribution made by people with dementia is, therefore, a fundamental element of the care encounter.

This notion of what we mean by contribution is, however, limited. As we move towards a situation whereby dementia and its diagnosis is increasingly shared and talked about within families, organisations and communities and ahead of what we might understand to be a caregiving context, there is scope to imagine a level of contribution to everyday life. One which moves away from passive receipt to active social citizenship (Bartlett and O'Connor 2010). Therefore alongside the notion of a contribution at an interpersonal level within a caring relationship is the progress towards genuine attempts to recognise the centrality of people who have dementia at a network or community level and enabling the "relational" and "social self" to flourish. NICE guidance draws attention to this aspect of community provisions with a clear emphasis on the role of agencies and organisations to help support and facilitate involvement (NICE 2013). NICE lists opportunities for continued contribution as volunteering, playing an active role in community activities and events, voting, raising awareness and offering peer support as well as being involved in intergenerational projects in schools. This list could be extended to include an active grand parenting role, paid work where appropriate, being involved in cultural activities and/or the church and local politics, nonetheless an integrated role is at the heart of the person's life. When considering the notion of contribution it is clear that the skills, knowledge, experiences, values, creative expression, wisdom and humour of the person with dementia can continue form a part of the lives of all community members (Norris and Woods 2016).

We propose that the notion of contribution should lie at the very heart of organisational and community values and for the purpose of this chapter propose a modified version of the senses framework (see Figure 3.2). This modified version is concerned with establishing contribution as an essential feature of organisational culture and values and that communities might sustain, via the third sector for instance. Furthermore, in keeping with all previous versions of the senses framework this version is also intended to be used with people with dementia, staff and family caregivers in mind.

Values in action

We have argued strongly here for the use of the notion of an "enriched environment" of care to help in being able to identify those environments where people with dementia, staff and family carers can be helped to experience care which is based on meaningful and trusting relationships. We have also suggested that the senses framework can help organisations to make sense of their own culture of care. In essence we feel that the senses framework is a useful heuristic device to use in practice for organisations to reflect upon and make judgements about their own operationalisation of the values that they hold. This chapter has also placed the notion of contribution at the centre of these organisational and community values. There is much work to be done to provide the opportunity for people who have dementia to contribute on all sorts of levels, not least the simple recognition of the part they play in care giving encounters. But we also believe that all of those who make a contribution should be recognised and have here provided the template for the consideration of the notion of contribution within the life of organisations and communities within a modified Senses Framework. The boundaries of care are shifting at all times and the potential for what we mean by an "enriched environment" may be very different in years to come. The values of caring organisations and communities, we suspect, should not change and should remain entirely focused on all of those affected by dementia and the contribution that they can make.

> **Security** – to ensure that the environment allows for people who have dementia, staff and family members to have their voices heard
>
> **Belonging** – to recognise that organisations are formed by communities of people with shared interests and goals, that organisational and community life is a joint, integrated venture
>
> **Continuity** – to seek to ensure that the life time skills and capacities of people with dementia, staff and family members are recognised and utilised to innovate and sustain a vibrant community life
>
> **Purpose** – to seek to ensure that the contribution of people who have dementia, staff or family members is meaningful to them, is consistent with their long term goals or aspirations
>
> **Achievement** – to create the opportunities for sustained contribution at all levels and to provide the support for this to make a difference
>
> **Significance** – to celebrate the contribution made by all within the care and wider community, to make it explicit and recognisable

Figure 3.2 Making a contribution via the senses framework

References

Adams, T. and Bartlett, R. (2003) *Dementia Care*. London: Arnold.

Baldwin, C., Capstick, A., Phinney, A., Purves, B., O'Connor, D. and Chaudhury, H. (2007) "Personhood". In *Tom Kitwood on Dementia: A Reader and Critical Commentary*. Maidenhead: Open University Press: 173–187.

Balfour, A. (2014) "Why should we be interested in supporting the couple relationship in dementia?" *Psychoanalytic Psychotherapy*, 28(3): 304–320.

Bartlett, R. and O'Connor, D. (2010)*Broadening the dementia debate: Towards social citizenship*. Bristol: The Policy Press.

Blood, I. (2013) *A Better Life: Valuing Our Later Years*. Joseph Rowntree Foundation: York.

Brooker, D. and Latham, I. (2016) *Person Centred Dementia Care: Making services better with the VIPS framework*. London: Jessica Kingsley Publishers.

Clarke, A. and Warren, L. (2007) Hopes, fears and expectations about the future: what do older people's stories tell us about active ageing? *Ageing & Society*, 27(4):465–488.

Dementia Action Alliance (2014) National Dementia Declaration for England. Available from: http://www.dementiaaction.org.uk/assets/0001/1915/National_Dementia_Declaration_for_England.pdf (accessed 3/3/2017).

Department of Health (2015) "Prime Minister's Challenge on Dementia 2020." London: Department of Health.

Dupuis, S.L., Gillies, J., Carson, J., Whyte, C., Genoe, R., Loiselle, L. and Sadler, L. (2011) "Moving beyond patient and client approaches: Mobilizing 'authentic partnerships' in dementia care, support and services." *Dementia: The International Journal of Social Research and Practice*, 11(4): 427–452.

Hellström, I., Nolan, M. and Lundh, U. (2007) "Sustaining 'couplehood': Spouses strategies for living positively with dementia." *Dementia: The International Journal of Social Research and Practice*, 6(3): 383–409.

Hughes, J. (2013) "'Y' feel me? How do we understand the person with dementia?" *Dementia: The International Journal of Social Research and Practice*, 12(3): 348–358.

Katz, J., Holland, C., Peace, S. and Taylor, E. (2011) *A Better Life - What Older People With High Support Needs Value*. York: Joseph Rowntree Foundation.

Kitwood, T. (1997) *Dementia Reconsidered: The person comes first*. Buckingham: Open University Press.

Marck, P. (1990) "Therapeutic Reciprocity: A caring phenomenon." *Advances in Nursing Science*, 13(1): 49–59.

McCormack, B. and McCance, T. (2010) *Person-centred Nursing: Theory & Practice*. Chichester: Wiley Blackwell.

Molyneaux, V., Butchard, S., Simpson, J. and Murray, C. (2012) "The Co-construction of Couplehood in Dementia." *Dementia: The International Journal of Social Research and Practice*, 11(4): 483–502.

Morhardt, D. and Spira, M. (2013) "From Person-Centered Care to Relational Centered Care." *Generations*, 8(3), 37–44.

NICE (National Institute for Health & Care Excellence) (2013) *Dementia: Independence & wellbeing*. London:NICE.

Nolan, M. R., Brown, J., Davies, S., Nolan, J. and Keady, J. (2006) "The Senses Framework: Improving Care for Older People Through a Relationship-Centred Approach." *Getting Research into Practice (GRiP) Report No 2*, University of Sheffield.

Norris, A. and Woods, B. (2016) "Spirituality and wisdom." In Clarke, C. and Wolverson, E. (Eds.) *Positive Psychology Approaches to Dementia*. London: Jessica Kingsley Publishers.

Roach, P., Keady, J. and Bee, P. (2012) "'It's easier just to separate them': practice constructions in the mental health care and support of younger people with dementia and their families." *Psychiatric & Mental Health Nursing*, 19(6): 555–562.

Robertson, J. M. (2014) Finding meaning in everyday life with dementia: A case study, *Dementia: The International Journal of Social Research and Practice*, 13(4): 525–543.

Rowe, J. and Kahn, R. (1997) "Successful Ageing." *The Gerontologist*, 37(4): 433–440.

Ryan, T., Nolan, M. R., Reid, D. and Enderby, P. (2008) "Using the Senses Framework to achieve relationship-centred dementia care services: a case example." *Dementia: The International Journal of Social Research and Practice*, 7(1): 71–93.

Tanner, D. (2010) *Managing the Ageing Experience: Learning from Older People.* Bristol: The Policy Press.

Toms, G., Clare, L., Nixon, J. and Quinn, C. (2015) "A systematic narrative review of support groups for people with dementia." *International Psychogeriatrics*, 27(9): 1439–1465.

Wiles, J., Wild, K., Kerse, N. & Allen, R. (2011) "Resilience from the point of view of older people: 'There's still life beyond a funny knee.'" *Social Science & Medicine*, 74: 416–424

WHO (2002) "Active Ageing: A Policy Framework." Available from: http://apps.who.int/iris/bit stream/10665/67215/1/WHO_NMH_NPH_02.8.pdf (accessed 3/3/2017).

Tresolini, C. P. and the Pew-Fetzer Task Force (1994) *Health Professions, Education and Relationship-centred Care.* San Francisco: Pew Fetzer Health Professions Commission.

Van Gennip, L. E., Pasman, R. W., Oosterveld-Vlug, M. G., Willems, D. L. and Onwuteaka-Philipsen, B. D. (2014) "How dementia affects personal dignity: A qualitative study of individuals with mild to moderate dementia." *Journals of Gerontology, Series B: Psychological and Social Sciences*, 71(3): 491–501.

Further Reading

Brooker, D. and Latham, I. (2015)*Person-centred dementia care: Making services better with the VIPS framework.* London: Jessica Kingsley Publishers.

Ryan, T. and Nolan, M. (2016) "Positive Psychology and Relational Dementia Care." In Clarke, C. & Wolverson, E. (eds.) *Positive Psychology Approaches to Dementia.* London: Jessica Kingsley Publishers.

4 Early diagnosis

Turning policy into practice

Stephen Lithgow and Robert Boyd

Introduction

In this chapter we will focus on the area of dementia diagnosis. We will consider the policy drivers to increase diagnosis rates and the push for earlier diagnosis. It will be shown that turning this aspect of dementia policy into practice can be challenging and that the diagnosis of dementia is a complicated and dynamic issue. It is one in which the interpretation of many factors is undertaken, and is a complex medical and social task.

Getting a diagnosis is important. It is the gateway to services and support. It can also provide a sense of understanding to the person with dementia and their carers, giving an explanation for the symptoms they may have been experiencing. Diagnosis can also be the start of a process where a person with dementia begins to make sense of the illness and plan for the future.

The diagnostic process itself is obviously an important aspect in determining early diagnosis. The role of guidance, medical training, knowledge and experience of dementia, use of assessment tools, access to scanning, and the role of the multi-disciplinary team all have a part to play. However, there are a range of barriers which influence levels of diagnosis and how early a diagnosis is made. The question of when, where, how or even if a diagnosis is made, is shaped by the following:

- Intrinsic factors. The willingness of a person with dementia to seek help.
- Policy factors. Policy drivers and how they are interpreted and implemented.
- Systematic factors. The ability of people with dementia to reach assessment for diagnosis. This includes pathways and other barriers.
- Interpretation of diagnosis from practitioner making the diagnosis. This includes the influence of the 'Timely versus Early' diagnosis debate.

Whilst the diagnostic process is central to the discussion, a study of dementia diagnosis needs to look more broadly and consider the complex influences at work before, during and after diagnosis.

Diagnosis and policy

Most dementia policy is now homogenous in approach. There is acknowledgement of the future increase in prevalence through modelling and a focus on increasing diagnosis rates (with an emphasis on earlier or timely diagnosis) and the redesigning and improving of services post diagnosis. In addition, policy looks to build knowledge, skills and capacity in the workforce, including unpaid carers and awareness raising in society in general.

The twin goals of increased diagnosis and earlier diagnosis should also be seen in the context of other aspects of dementia policy. For example, increasing awareness and reducing stigma could have a longer-term influence on diagnosis by encouraging people to talk more about dementia, feel less fearful and be more willing to seek help. Other policy aspects such as the development of post diagnosis support, emphasise the benefits of earlier diagnosis and could encourage people to come forward.

Establishing prevalence and incidence

An important starting point in implementing policy such as increasing diagnosis rates is to firstly gauge an accurate picture of prevalence (existing dementia in a population) and incidence (expected new diagnosis in a population). How do we establish how many people are expected to have dementia in a city or country and how do we know what percentage of this group have been given a diagnosis? This data is essential if services are to be planned properly and future service demands accurately projected.

Box 4.1 Case study: Dementia incidence in Scotland (November 2016)

Incidence: Initial data gathered from early post-diagnosis service provision in Scotland suggested higher than expected incidence levels of dementia.

Incidence had been calculated previously using an estimate obtained from analysis taken from a Medical Research Council-funded study, "The Incidence of Dementia in England and Wales: Findings from Five Identical Sites of the MRC CFA Study" (Matthews and Brayne 2005). Information Services Division at NHS National Services Scotland noted that: "Limitations of the study were of the assumption of a patient's survival time post-diagnosis and the number of individuals dying after developing dementia before receiving a formal diagnosis". Further study of 'real life' data" from three NHS Health Boards providing support found that dementia incidence was underestimated by 50%. This new work provided a more rigorous evaluation of dementia incidence in Scotland "Estimated and projected diagnosis rates for dementia in Scotland; 2014–2020" (Scottish Government 2016).

Another prominent issue is establishing the stage of dementia at diagnosis. Firstly, this needs to be captured and recorded if we are to establish progress on the policy goal of increasing early diagnosis. Secondly, the stage of dementia at diagnosis impacts on the benefit of post diagnosis supports and on how post diagnosis services are delivered. For example, later stage diagnosis leaves less scope for work around areas such as supported self-management or the ability to plan ahead.

Establishing the stage of dementia is not an exact science. It is linked to cognitive assessment which may be in turn influenced by issues such as sensory impairment, tiredness, depression, education and cultural sensitivity. Ideally a comprehensive assessment should be undertaken (NICE 2016).

Negative aspects of early diagnosis

Although policy reflects a view that increased diagnosis levels is a positive outcome, it is important to consider the possible benefits a diagnosis brings to the person with dementia and their families.

The assumption that giving a diagnosis is good needs to be seen in the context of what happens after the diagnosis is made. Without practical and emotional help in the form of post diagnosis support, the real benefit of giving a diagnosis is questionable. In addition people may not wish to accept support even if available as they may feel they do not need the service at that stage. That is their choice.

For those not receiving support following a diagnosis, could giving a diagnosis be more harmful than not giving one? Giving a diagnosis poses an age-old ethical question associated with beneficence versus non-maleficence. Is a diagnosis of dementia with no follow up support an example of a diagnosis with ineffective treatment? Studies of dementia carers suggest that early diagnosis can be more beneficial to help caregivers adapt but that these benefits can be outweighed if little overall support is offered. Early diagnosis alone is therefore not necessarily beneficial. It needs to be followed up with effective post diagnosis support that includes the carer and which can be accessed when the person with dementia feels will be beneficial

Sometimes a diagnosis is made but not always disclosed. A carer may be told, but not the person with dementia. Here, practitioners are weighing up the pros and cons of a diagnosis in terms of disclosure. In relation to rights, the person with dementia also has the right not to know, but this is different from a diagnosis being withheld. However, in terms of rights is the person given a diagnosis not entitled to the same access to treatment/support someone with another illness may receive, such as cancer?

Box 4.2 Dementia diagnosis for individuals

Compare a diagnosis of dementia given to two people with dementia with similar needs. One lives in an area with access to effective post diagnosis support and the other has no support offered. What are the possible outcomes of receiving a diagnosis for the individuals?

It should also be considered that there are some negative aspects of getting a diagnosis of dementia even with the right kind of support. The person may feel labelled by getting a diagnosis, or be dealing with the stigma that still exists in society. Personal fear of dementia is still a major issue for many older people. Jennings and Foley (2014) found that diagnosis could potentially have a negative impact on the doctor-patient relationship. Ultimately, anyone with a diagnosis of dementia may still experience aspects of Kirkwood's Malignant Social Psychology, such as infantilisation and exclusion. Yes, many people do live a good life with dementia but it is unwise to ignore the negative aspects that still prevail in some parts of society, despite public campaigns.

As diagnosis rates increase so do the demands on the resources associated with the diagnostic process and post diagnosis support. Increasingly a multi-agency approach including health and social care integration and the third sector are working together. Where and how a diagnosis is made directly influences its cost. For example there are additional costs of making a diagnosis in a specialist service rather than in primary care. In some areas of the UK memory clinics (sometimes known as memory assessment services) are also on the increase. There is a general acknowledgment that this increase in the UK came about after the inception of cholinesterase inhibitors (Meeuwsen et al. 2012).

Memory clinics

The Department of Health (2006) recommended that memory assessment services should be the preferred point of referral for all people with a possible diagnosis of dementia. There is no precise definition for what constitutes a memory clinic or the level of multidisciplinary involvement, but there is a general acceptance that there should be team approach and the diagnosis should be given along with information and support for the person and family. This differs from the 1970s when memory clinics began in the USA as part of academic research initiatives looking at Alzheimer's disease, often for drug trials (Beese 2000). Similarly in the 1980s memory clinics were set up in the UK primarily to gather information for research purposes, although possibly not to the same extent as in the USA. Initially they were criticised for being medically oriented, offering little in the way of social support. Recent literature indicates newer clinics tend to operate on a multidisciplinary model, involving assessment, investigation, and information giving as recommended by NICE (2016).

However, types of memory clinics appear to differ in specialties, the exact protocol applied, time spent on assessment, and advice offered (Cantley and Smith 2007). For example, the initial assessment visit can vary from one to seven hours

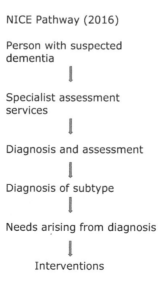

NICE Pathway (2016)

Person with suspected dementia

Specialist assessment services

Diagnosis and assessment

Diagnosis of subtype

Needs arising from diagnosis

Interventions

Figure 4.1 NICE pathway

and, while some only take direct referrals from within the NHS, other clinics tend to focus on a self-referral basis. Some clinics offer support and counselling as part of their service, and others refer on to other agencies. Some offer memory retraining and anxiety management within their clinics and psychosocial educational programmes. Some also offer pre-diagnostic counselling, support groups, psychotherapy, and cognitive behavioural therapy. Moreover, some clinics routinely follow up all their patients, whilst some follow up only uncertain cases or selected diagnostic cases (Szymczynska et al. 2011). For example, some protocols state that people with Alzheimer's disease who have been prescribed cholinesterase inhibitors should be seen regularly to be monitored whilst taking the medication. This often leads to additional therapeutic interventions and support (possibly more useful than the medication). In contrast, those with a diagnosis of vascular dementia not requiring medication were previously discharged from the memory services as they did not require "treatment". However currently, the development of post diagnosis support policy does not differentiate between types of dementia (Scottish Government 2013).

NICE (2016) does not specify exactly what memory clinics should offer, but developed a pathway allowing teams to have a flexible approach to be adopted. However, this flexible approach could lead to inequalities in support. The term 'postcode lottery' is often used to describe services for people with dementia.

The growing development of post diagnosis support (PDS) services and dementia-friendly communities are seen as important supports to those who receive a diagnosis. Post diagnosis models have been designed to support people at the earlier stages of getting a diagnosis. However in practice, the stage of diagnosis is made has an important impact on how post diagnosis services are delivered.

Box 4.3 Case study: Scotland

Scotland provides an interesting case study of dementia policy which aims to increase diagnosis rates whilst providing a national post diagnosis support (PDS) guarantee. In Scotland, everyone with a new diagnosis of dementia is guaranteed support for at least a year from a dementia link worker, who will work with them and their carers around a five-pillar approach developed by Alzheimer Scotland. This includes the provision of information, peer support, planning for legal issues, planning ahead using a personal plan and keeping connected (Alzheimer Scotland 2011).

In Scotland, the data suggests that there still remain challenges with an early diagnosis PDS model, only around 50% of new diagnosis of dementia made each year are in the early stages. This leaves many people with more advanced dementia who will still be offered post diagnosis support. This can mean an opportunity is missed to carry out specific earlier stage dementia work. As a result of later diagnosis, link workers appear to be adapting their work. This can mean less "light touch" work and more work with carers or health and social care supports. This has meant a much broader than anticipated range of dementia in the field of post diagnosis support. The key message is that early diagnosis is still not yet the norm.

Barriers to diagnosis

There are many reasons why a diagnosis of dementia can take time to make and much of the literature around dementia diagnosis relates to barriers. It has been estimated that it may take up to two and a half years from thinking something is wrong, to talking about it to first contacting a health professional. Then further time can elapse before diagnosis is made (Chrisp et al. 2012). Partly it is intrinsic, partly systematic, but we will also see the personal interpretation by the medical practitioner may also play a part.

Intrinsic barriers

Individuals and caregivers may be reluctant to seek a diagnosis due to stigma and fear. There may be denial of symptoms by the person with dementia and their family (Greenway-Crombie et al. 2012). There can be fear of a loss of independence, such as losing a driving licence. A lack of awareness of the signs and symptoms of dementia may also act as a barrier. When a person lives alone they often lack the support or view of a loved one to encourage them to seek help. People with dementia and their families may not be sure when they should seek help. Some may think the symptoms of dementia such as short-term memory loss are just a part of getting old.

Systematic barriers

Some barriers are systematic, including a lack of support, time and financial constraints for GPs. Koch et al. (2010) identified GP uncertainty around diagnosis, disclosing the diagnosis and confidence in making it. They may also be influenced by therapeutic nihilism, feeling little can be done. GPs often feel they need better training, including how to break bad news.

   Health inequalities exist around diagnosis as they do with other health conditions. In more deprived areas people with dementia and their carers may be less well informed about support services or less likely to push for a diagnosis. Age can influence earlier diagnosis, with Young Onset Dementia typically taking longer to diagnose. Similarly, marginalised groups, such as the homeless and those in prisons are less likely to be diagnosed early. In other settings such as nursing homes it is thought that new diagnosis is rarely made although up to 90% of residents may have dementia (Lithgow et al. 2012).

Interpretation of diagnosis: timely versus early

Separating early stage dementia from Mild Cognitive Impairment can be difficult. National dementia strategies often focus on early diagnosis and finding people with dementia, in some cases before there're are any obvious symptoms. For example in England, policy has rightly or wrongly influenced the introduction of case finding in high risk groups – including people over 75 years of age, as age is the strongest risk factor for dementia – and those with high vascular risk, Parkinson's disease, and learning disabilities (Robinson et al. 2015). The policy comprises proactive screening for signs of early stage dementia in patients who may not have symptoms, in general hospitals, primary care and community setting. There is little evidence that such initiatives, which predominantly lead to increased referrals to specialist memory services and clinic, are cost effective or whether they are distressing to patients (Robinson et al. 2015). While there are no specific blood tests or indicators for the majority of dementia subtypes at the moment, how 'early' would we want to diagnose pre-dementia should such tests become available? Moreover, whilst there is no cure or treatments to prevent the disease process, would people with a predisposition want to know? (Cuijpers and van Lente 2015)

The report of the Nuffield Council on Bioethics (2009) debates this issue from an ethical standpoint, arguing that there is a "distinction between early and timely diagnosis" and that if a person's wellbeing is not enhanced by receiving a potential diagnosis, the pros and cons need to be carefully considered.

In trying to define a timely diagnosis, Dhedhi et al. (2014) state that this is: "range of nuanced balancing judgements, often negotiated with patients and their families with detailed attention to a particular context". In this instance GPs are attempting to gauge the right time to give a diagnosis. As a result timely diagnosis is not necessarily a snapshot in time, it is more cumulative and collective, where the consequences are considered. It is argued that a timely diagnosis is more beneficial for a person with dementia, healthcare professional and society than early diagnosis (De Lepeleire et al. 2008). There is a recognition that one size does not fit all, it is more about an appropriate time for the person and their family (Fox et al. 2013). Hansen et al. (2008) note that dementia is seen from an "holistic viewpoint" where "GPs assess diagnosis within the broader context of patient's lives."

With a timely diagnosis Cahill et al. (2006) note the patient's perception of diagnosis is considered. Bunn et al. (2012) acknowledge that early diagnosis and intervention is seen as a priority but practitioners are concerned with the effects of giving earlier diagnosis. These were identified into three key themes: (i) pathways through diagnosis and impact on role, identity and relationships; (ii) revolving conflicts to accommodate a diagnosis, including the acceptability of support; (iii) strategies and support to minimise the impact of dementia.

Conclusion

Diagnosis of dementia remains a contemporary issue and one of the main challenges for the 21st century. Policies and strategies push for an early diagnosis, linked to the development of post diagnosis support and advanced care planning. However, turning any policy into practice can be challenging and the area of diagnosis of dementia is no exception to this. The diagnosis of dementia is a complicated and dynamic issue. More recently the term "timely" diagnosis has emerged, indicating that the drive for early diagnosis may not always be in everyone's best interests. This subjective and nuanced approach is potentially a challenge for policy makers who have tended to focus on early diagnosis, rather than the broader context and consequences of the diagnosis.

More traditional services such as memory clinics are evolving to offer a more holistic and person-centred approach to diagnosis. Similarly, post diagnosis support is now focusing on a social model with service often provided by third sector organisations.

Influences before, during and after diagnosis are continuing to be addressed by policy makers, and there is a recognition that a broad range of organisations and stakeholders need to work together to support the person with dementia. Ultimately, the diagnosis of dementia can mean a myriad of different individual experiences and responses shaped by abroad range of often external factors.

References

Alzheimer Scotland (2011) "5 Pillars Model of Post Diagnostic support." Available from: http://www.alzscot.org/campaigning/five_pillars.

Beese, R. (2000) "Memory clinics: a potential 'one stop shop' for services." *Journal of Dementia Care*, 8(2), 35–37.

Bunn, F., Goodman, C., Sworn, K., Rait, G., Brayne, C., Robinson, L., McNeilly, E. and Iliffe, S. (2012) "Psychosocial factors that shape patient and carer experiences of dementia diagnosis and treatment: a systematic review of qualitative studies." *PLoS Med* 9(10): e1001331. doi:10.1371/journal.pmed.1001331.

Cahill, S., Clark, M., Walsh, C., O'Connell, M., Lawlor, B. (2006) "Dementia in primary care: the first survey of Irish practitioners." *International Journal of Geriatric Psychiatry*, 21(4): 319–324.

Cantley, C. and Smith, M. (2007) "Getting on with living: a guide to developing dementia support services." Mental Health Foundation. Available from: https://www.mentalhealth.org.uk/publications/getting-living.

Chrisp, T.A.C., Tabberer, S., Thomas, B.D. and Goddard, W.A. (2012) "Dementia early diagnosis: triggers, supports and constraints affecting the decision to engage with the health care system." *Aging & Mental Health*, 16(5): 559–565.

Cuijpers, Y. and van Lente, H. (2015) "Early diagnostics and Alzheimer's disease: beyond 'cure' and 'care'." *Technological Forecasting and Social Change*, 93: 54–67. doi:10.1016/j.techfore.2014.03.006.

De Lepeleire, J., Wind, A.W., Iliffe, S., Moniz-Cook, E.D., Wilcock, J., Gonzalez, V.M., Derksen, E., Gianelli, M.V., Vernooij-Dassen, M. and Interdem Group (2008) "The primary care diagnosis of dementia in Europe: an analysis using multidisciplinary, multinational expert groups." *Aging & Mental Health*, 12(5): 568–576.

Dhedhi, S.A., Swinglehurst, D. and Russell, J. (2014) "'Timely' diagnosis of dementia: what does it mean? A narrative analysis of GPs' accounts." *BMJ Open*, 4: e004439. doi:10.1136/bmjopen-2013004439.

Fox, C., Lafortune, L., Boustani, M. and Brayne, C. (2013) "The pros and cons of early diagnosis in dementia." *British Journal of General Practice*, 63(612): 510–512.

Greenway-Crombie, A., Snow, P., Disler, P., Davis, S. and Pond, D. (2012) "Influence of rurality on diagnosing dementia in Australian general practice." *Australian Journal of Primary Health*, 18(3): 178–184.

Hansen, E.C., Hughes, C., Routley, G. and Robinson, A.L. (2008) "General practitioners' experiences and understandings of diagnosing dementia: Factors impacting on early diagnosis." *Social Science & Medicine*, 67(11): 1776–1783.

Jennings, A. and Foley, T. (2014), "The barriers to diagnosing dementia in primary care: A qualitative GP registrar perspective." 62nd Annual and Scientific Meeting of the Irish Gerontological Society, Galway, Ireland. 9–11 October 2014. *Irish Journal of Medical Science*, 183(7) SUPPL. 1: S347.

KochT., Iliffe, S. and E.V.I.D.E.M.E.D. (2010) "Rapid appraisal of barriers to the diagnosis and management of patients with dementia in primary care: a systematic review." *BMC Family Practice*, 11: 52.

Lithgow, S., Jackson, G. and Browne, D. (2012) "Estimating the prevalence of dementia: cognitive screening in Glasgow nursing homes." *International Journal of Geriatric Psychiatry*, 27(8): 785–791. doi:10.1002/gps.2784.

Matthews, F., Brayne, C. and Medical Research Council Cognitive Function and Ageing Study Investigators (2005) "The Incidence of Dementia in England and Wales: Findings from the Five Identical Sites of the MRC CFA Study." *PLoS Med* 2(8): e193.

Meeuwsen, E.J., Melis, R.J., Van Der Aa, G.C., Golüke-Willemse, G.A., De Leest, B.J., Van Raak, F.H., Schölzel-Dorenbos, C.J., Verheijen, D.C., Verhey, F.R. and Visser, M.C. (2012) "Effectiveness of dementia follow-up care by memory clinics or general practitioners: Randomised controlled trial." *British Medical Journal* 344: e3086. doi:10.1136/bmj.e3086.

NICE (National Institute for Health and Clinical Excellence and Social care for Excellence) (2016) "NICE clinical guideline. Dementia: supporting people with health and social care." Available from: http://www.nice.org.uk/CG42.

Nuffield Council on Bioethics (2009) Dementia: ethical issues. http://nuffieldbioethics.org/project/dementia.

Robinson, L., Tang, E. and Taylor, J.P. (2015) "Dementia: timely diagnosis and early intervention." *British Medical Journal*, June 16(350): h3029. doi:10.1136/bmj.h3029.

Scottish Government (2016) "Estimated and Projected Diagnosis Rates for Dementia in Scotland 2014–20120." Available from: http://www.gov.scot/Publications/2016/12/9363/1.

Scottish Government (2013) "Scotland's National Dementia Strategy. 2010–20123." Available from: http://www.gov.scot/Topics/Health/Services/MentalHealth/Dementia/DementiaStrategy1316.

Szymczynska, P., Innes, A., Mason, A. and Stark, C. (2011) "A Review of Diagnostic Process and Postdiagnostic Support for People with Dementia in Rural Areas." *Journal of Primary Care & Community Health*, 2: 262–276.

Further reading

NHS Choices. "How to get a dementia diagnosis." Available from: https://www.nhs.uk/conditions/dementia/diagnosis/.

NHS Choices. "Testing for diagnosing dementia." Available from: https://www.nhs.uk/conditions/dementia/diagnosis-tests/.

National Institute for Clinical Excellence. "Dementia Diagnosis and Assessment." Available from: https://pathways.nice.org.uk/pathways/dementia/dementia-diagnosis-and-assessment.

Alzheimer's Disease International. "Diagnosis." Available from: https://www.alz.co.uk/info/diagnosis.

NHS England. (2015) "Dementia Diagnosis and Management. A brief pragmatic resource for general practitioners." Available from: https://www.england.nhs.uk/wp-content/uploads/2015/01/dementia-diag-mng-ab-pt.pdf.

Alzheimer's Research UK. "Getting Diagnosed." Available from: https://www.alzheimersresearchuk.org/about-dementia/helpful-information/getting-diagnosed/.

World Health Organisation (WHO) (2017) "Global action plan on the public health response to dementia 2017–2025." Available from: http://www.who.int/mental_health/neurology/dementia/action_plan_2017_2025/en/.

5 Where does dementia sit in modern society?

Karen Watchman

Introduction

Attitudes towards people with dementia have changed in the 21st century. We now have a greater emphasis on self-advocacy and inclusion, with the mantra "nothing about us without us" being adopted from disability advocates of the 1990s. This chapter considers the changing landscape and the policy shifts that have reframed how we think about dementia, particularly the development and implementation of national dementia plans or strategies. However, not everyone with dementia has been affected by this changing paradigm and instead we continue to witness marginalisation within some minority populations. Much is said about human rights internationally yet we do not always have the human right to be heard or to "have a voice". Organisations such as the Scottish and European Dementia Working Groups and Dementia Alliance International strive and advocate for improved services for people with dementia. However, there are still minority groups who remain silent.

Current knowledge

Many minority groups are not identified in national dementia policies, and so may not receive the services available for others. Here we discuss some of these.

The UK has its oldest ever population of prisoners with dementia with the number estimated to increase from 4,100 in 2015 to 5,500 in 2020. Many lesbian, gay or bisexual or transgender (LGBT) residents in care homes are afraid to be open about their sexuality. The word dementia does not translate into some languages, with low awareness and high stigma existing among black and minority ethnic communities. At the same time the current estimate of nearly 25,000 people with dementia from BME communities in England and Wales is expected to grow to nearly 50,000 by 2026 and over 172,000 by 2051. This represents almost a seven-fold increase in 40 years, compared to just over a two-fold increase in the numbers of people with dementia across the whole UK population in the same time period. It is estimated that at least one in three people with Down's syndrome over the age of 50 will have dementia, often coinciding with the poor health or death of their parent and primary carer.

There is a significant lack of evidence from which to develop support for such populations of people as dementia becomes more advanced and increased support is required.

Prisoners

With a growing population of older people in prisons it is no surprise that the number of people with dementia will also increase. But are we training prison staff to identify the changes that may indicate the onset, especially in an environment where withdrawal, communication difficulties, apathy and changes in behaviour are commonly experienced? After all, this is a role that typically expects staff to take a more punitive stance of punishing aggressive inmates rather than evaluating them for Alzheimer's disease.

An increase in the number of people with dementia, men and women, in prison also raises a further neglected 21st-century challenge of prisoners' families; whether this is due to more older people being admitted to prison as first offenders which leaves more older partners at home, some of whom will have dementia themselves; or ageing parents who have an adult child in prison. Long-term prisoners may be even more susceptible to dementia due to a combination of risk factors: poor education, and higher rates of hypertension, diabetes, depression, substance abuse and head injuries. Visiting areas are exactly the kind of noisy environments that we warn people with dementia to avoid. Long-term prisoners with dementia, despite failing short-term memory, may vividly recall the crime that led to their incarceration, whilst others recognise family members in reflections rather than themselves, some of whom may have also been involved in the crime, either as a partner or a victim. All of which, combined with the lack of prison based palliative care programmes, adds up to a cauldron of triggers and resulting behaviours that challenge both the staff and other prisoners.

The Mental Health Foundation made a number of recommendations in their 2013 report: that a cognitive screen be taken on all new arrivals over the age of 50; that basic dementia training is provided for all prison staff; that clearer referral procedures are put in place to speed up the process of diagnosis, and that prisons should be physically adapted to accommodate prisoners with dementia, for example clearer signage. A prison in New York took a more radical approach. Faced with overwhelming numbers of prisoners with dementia at California Men's Colony it is prisoners themselves who are being trained to support others with dementia in some activities of daily living. Although much of their approach appears to be reactive to behavioural challenges and potentially leaving other prisoners in difficult situations, other more positive initiatives have been introduced such as a 'slow eaters' table and advocacy at health appointments, placing dementia and cognitive impairment higher on the prison agenda.

Box 5.1 Discussion point

There will come a point when the advanced stage of dementia renders prisoners incapable of committing further crimes. Do prisoners merely serve a symbolic role in detailing individuals with dementia or, as has been the case with individuals in an advanced stage of cancer, should prison be deemed inappropriate for prisoners with dementia?

LGBT

Many LGBT people believe that should they require support services in the future those available will not fully meet their needs, especially in a care home context where there is a feeling that individuals may face prejudice and discrimination if staff know of their sexuality. Historically, LGBT people have not had their relationships legally recognised. The social and historical context is that many, especially individuals who are now older, will have lived with oppression and inequality. Applying person-centred concepts has become the norm and the expectation in provision of dementia care, however this means moving away from the assumption of similarities between people. Instead, they call for an increased awareness of particular challenges that LGBT people face. This is consistent with a study in the North East of England where focus group members did not want to be treated the same as other people with dementia, they wanted their individual identity as a lesbian or gay person to be recognised. Trans people face different social and body issues: there is anecdotal evidence of services being denied, prevention of cross dressing and physical violence when people are identified as trans in a care home setting. Cognitive difficulties associated with dementia may cause specific challenges for trans people in maintaining gender identity. When this is combined with gender-related medical issues, such as prostate cancer, it can lead to confusion and distress in self-care. Age UK (2015) noted the importance of respecting privacy in terms of wearing a hair piece, shaving and the type of clothing worn. A further 21st-century challenge is the increasingly popular use of reminiscence therapy that may lead to recall of a time when the person was younger and lived their life in a different gender role, although research related to sexual diversity and dementia is sparse. It is clear that there are additional concerns that must be faced when providing dementia care whether in residential, day or home care settings.

Box 5.2 Discussion point

The last LGBT person I dealt with in this situation was about two years ago…. He went into residential care. Then immediately he went straight back into the closet.

(Peel and McDaid 2015)

Consider why this may have happened, read your national dementia strategy or plan and consider how far this supports staff to provide better care for LGBT people.

Learning disability

One in three people over the age of 50 who have Down's syndrome are estimated to have dementia. Yet, with life expectancy only recently extending beyond the age of 60 for people with Down's syndrome, this leaves the potential for a period of ageing with increased cognitive impairment whilst not "fitting" into aged care services which are typically for those aged over 65, or into learning disability services where the long-term focus in the UK is on independence, self-advocacy and informed choice. For some, pre-existing non-verbal communication methods, poor pain detection, increased sensory impairment and lack of accurate diagnosis of dementia mean that this group also stand out as presenting with new challenges in the 21st century requiring a different, yet related, response to the populations discussed earlier. For example, people with a learning disability are more likely to have physical health conditions that are not managed well. These conditions can either mask the early symptoms of dementia leading to a delayed diagnosis, or are assumed to be associated with dementia when in fact they are due to a different treatable condition. Examples in people with Down's syndrome include: hypothyroidism, effects of obesity, sleep apnoea or ear infections caused by small ear canal and large adenoids. There is also increased propensity to self-talk; private speech aloud which is generally viewed as adaptive and a coping mechanism in people with Down's syndrome rather than a concern.

Whilst there is more attention paid now to diagnosis and to understand changes in behaviour that may indicate dementia, we still do not have accurate data of the incidence of Down's syndrome, let alone Down's syndrome and dementia. Quantitative research has focused on clinical areas around brain function and diagnosis whilst qualitative studies have looked at early signs of dementia and wellbeing of carers. Despite advances generally, research continues to neglect the issue of advanced dementia in this population; there remains a deficit of tools that help to identify when someone is moving to their last days of life or that can determine quality of life in people with a learning disability and dementia. Existing tools for people with dementia use measures that assume marriage or long-term relationship, employment and financial dependency, whereas tools for people with a learning disability generally include maintenance of community based activities that may not be a long-term quality of life indicator as dementia progresses. Where people with a learning disability and dementia live tends to be different too. Many people in the UK live in the family home with parents or a sibling and the onset of dementia often comes at a time when older parents are often coping with their own multimorbidity or even dementia, and siblings may have their own children and are often in employment.

Box 5.3 Discussion point

What are the key differences in how dementia is experienced by people with, and without a learning disability?

BME

Within BME groups we see reports of a higher risk of misdiagnosis and delayed care. Fewer than half of the population receive a diagnosis despite increased risk of diabetes, heart disease and high blood pressure, common risk factors among Asian and black Caribbean communities. Predominantly, within the BME community, fewer referrals from GPs reach a psychiatrist or neurologist. This contributes to misdiagnosis, inappropriate treatment and ultimately a heavier commitment for families and society to manage.

The cognitive tests that are carried out in the GP clinic compare performance to the majority White British population norms meaning that a perceived or actual cultural bias exists that may limit the value of the assessment process for some BME older people. Consequently, the lack of BME-specific norms is considered to be a barrier in making an accurate diagnosis of dementia.

Many communities may not be prepared for the changes which are occurring and that it may be difficult to reconcile the needs and expectations of older people with those of their families: for example, older people may have expectations of being cared for by extended family, whilst families may be in the difficult position of juggling caring responsibilities. It is a commonly held perception that BME communities "look after their own", living in extended families and providing support to older family members. However, such trends are changing with an increasing number of people in BME communities living alone; indeed this was highlighted as early as the 2011 census in the UK.

Some South Asian and European languages do not have a word for dementia and the Arabic translation is related to insanity. Negative perceptions of dementia are compounded by such poorly-translated terms. In other ethnic groups such as the Irish and Jewish population, there is a demographically-older population so with the link between age and dementia prevalence is likely to be higher. This presents challenges for providers of dementia services if they have not worked with cultural groups previously or if their commissioning processes do not take into account the major shifts in demographics currently taking place.

Box 5.4 Discussion point

There is a commonly held perception that BME communities "look after their own". How relevant is this in the 21st century with an increase in social isolation and loneliness among older people generally?

Implications for dementia care in modern society – where can we do things better?

Two of the groups discussed in this chapter, people with a learning disability and LGBT people, come under the umbrella of the Equality Act 2010 that protects from discrimination. However, prisoners and other populations not automatically covered by this legislation, such as the travelling community (unless there is a young onset diagnosis or co-existent disability), are trailing even further behind in terms of inclusion in policy or dementia strategies, and are not protected from unlawful discrimination or disadvantage. So how does this sit with competing priorities in the field of dementia care? Literature tells us that key priority issues in 21st century dementia care vary widely from national to localised; a GP report stated that their priorities were around diagnosis and training of GPs (Robinson and Cook 2014). The Alzheimer's Society (2013) identified integrated care as being a recent and crucial issue with a challenge being to overcome separate systems including record keeping and funding and the challenge of professionals working in silos. A Dementia and Equalities Group in Scotland (NHS Scotland 2016) identified four general themes of: awareness raising, the requirement for robust services and support pathways, appropriate skills and knowledge, and the need for further research. Yet it is apparent that mainstream research into dementia does not always include ethnic data, for example, the State of the Nation report in the UK (Department of Health 2013) has geographical breakdowns of diagnosis but no breakdown by different ethnic groups. This leaves the question of how we bring together the diversity among each of the populations discussed, and others, whilst still recognising the individuality in each diagnosis.

The World Health Organisation's report on Dementia: A Public Health Priority (WHO 2012) called for the development and adoption of national dementia plans or strategies to guide public policy and set development goals for services, supports, advocacy, and research related to dementia. Whilst there are currently 30 such plans in existence or in development across Europe, the total figure of only 81 worldwide suggests many countries have not yet adopted their first plan (Alzheimer's Europe 2015). Those that have a plan paid minimal attention to groups experiencing additional discrimination due to their marginalised status. To continue with learning disability as an example, Gardner (2016) conducted a survey of 79 dementia plans or strategies finding that only approximately 37% mentioned adults with a learning disability.

It should be noted that although some countries have yet to develop a national plan or strategy, a small number are on to their second, or in the case of Scotland, their third. Attention should be paid to changes in second and subsequent plans that recognise this development with an increased recognition, albeit in a limited manner, of the needs of marginalized populations in relation to dementia care as shown below.

> **Box 5.5 Key point: Progressive inclusion of people with a learning disability in national plans – Norway**
>
> In Norway's first dementia plan, people with a learning disability were not mentioned at all. In the second there is a distinct section with the clear recommendations that support models identified in national dementia plans should also be adapted to people with a learning disability.
>
> (Ministry of Health and Care Services 2015).

> **Box 5.6 Key point: Progressive inclusion of people with a learning disability in national plans – Scotland**
>
> In Scotland, the first dementia plan (Scottish Government 2010) made reference to the link between Down syndrome and dementia, while the second (Scottish Government 2013) made a specific commitment to seek further information that will inform the third strategy due in 2017.

> **Box 5.7 Key point: Progressive inclusion of people with a learning disability in national plans – USA**
>
> In the USA, the annual updates to the National Plan to Address Alzheimer's Disease stemming from the National Alzheimer's Project Act (2018) progressively have increased mention of learning disability since the Plan's first iteration in 2012.

Overall, this raises two important issues; firstly, to consider if this gradual increase in the meaningful inclusion of people with a learning disability in some national plans can be applied to LGBT, BME and prison populations. It serves to make the strategy and any associated recommendations for dementia-related training and awareness raising, immediately relevant for staff in supporting organisations. We need to consider if the lack of specific inclusion of other groups contribute to their further marginalisation as families affected and support staff do not see immediate relevance or how the strategy may also be applied to the individuals they support.

A more fundamental issue however is that the examples from Norway, Scotland and the USA show that the national dementia plan or strategy is not a static document. Each has developed with an increase in representation of people from minority populations, often with specific recommendations that has fed directly into the next strategy. So where does this leave dementia in modern society? Whilst no one dementia plan or strategy will work for a different country, the influence in planning or development groups for future strategies by marginalised populations or their chosen advocates can only serve to facilitate inclusion of typically quiet voices in 21st-century dementia care such as those representing prisoner, LGBT, learning disability and BME populations. Incidence of dementia will continue to increase, with a rise in the number of people undoubtedly challenging the acute, residential, community and home care sectors. The need to respond to the complexities of dementia among competing priorities has never been more prominent.

The increased focus in the 21st century on non-pharmacological advances should be embraced for the opportunity it affords all people affected by dementia to celebrate cultural and religious preferences, for example within reminiscence or life story work. Implementation of national dementia plans or strategies, provided they are regularly revised rather than static, one-off, documents provide further opportunity for marginalised groups to have a voice in planning groups and as part of the consultation process, all of which should be applauded. Yet, alongside this, the stigma and discrimination experienced by many individuals and populations on a day-to-day basis is continuing. Higher level policy or strategy implementation will only be effective if this is reinforced at ground level; if issues affecting specific groups appear in professional and post-qualifying training and education, if we identify accurate incidence and prevalence figures of dementia among marginalised groups and if we strive to include representatives of such populations at all stages of service planning and development. Without this, the gap between positive 21st-century developments seen in many countries of policy and strategy directives, and the day-to-day requirements of dementia care by prisoners, people with a learning disability, LGBT people and BME communities will remain unmet and will continue unchallenged.

Box 5.8 Discussion points

- Diagnosis rates among BME communities, people with a learning disability, older LGBT individuals and prisoners suggest clarity is needed in assessment and diagnostic pathways. How appropriate is the diagnosis process for the groups included in this chapter and how can we make improvements?
- How many different information styles or formats are you able to access about dementia, for example, translated or pictorial and how are these made available to groups who may benefit from it?

References

Age UK. (2015) *Lesbian, gay, bisexual or transgender: Planning for later life.* London: Age UK.

Alzheimer Europe National Dementia Strategies. (2016) "National Dementia Strategies." Available from: http://www.alzheimer-europe.org/Policy-in-Practice2/National-Dementia-Strategies.

Alzheimer's Society. (2013) *Consultation response to the Kings Fund: The future of health and social care.* London, UK: Alzheimer's Society.

Department of Health. (2013) *Dementia A state of the nation report on dementia care and support in England.* London: Department of Health.

Gardner, S.O. (2016) "Intellectual and developmental disabilities and dementia in national and sub-national dementia plans." Available from: https://www.alz.co.uk/alzheimer-plans/small-papers-on-national-and-sub-national-dementia-plans.

National Alzheimer's Project Act. (2018) Available from: https://aspe.hhs.gov/national-alzheimers-project-act.

Peel, E. and McDaid, S. (2015) "'Over the Rainbow' Lesbian, Gay, Bisexual and Trans People and Dementia Project Summary Report." Available from: https://dementiavoices.org.uk/wp-content/uploads/2015/03/Over-the-Rainbow-LGBTDementia-Report.pdf.

Robinson, L. and Cook, J. (2014) "Dementia care in primary care: a priority for 21st century GPs." *Clinical News* (May). Available from: http://www.rcgp.org.uk/-/media/Files/CIRC/Dementia/RCGP-Dementia-care-in-primary-care-May-2014.ashx?la=en

Scottish Government. (2010) *Scotland's National Dementia Strategy.* Edinburgh: Scottish Government. Available from: http://www.gov.scot/Resource/Doc/324377/0104420.pdf. Published 2010.

Scottish Government. (2013) *Scotland's National Dementia Strategy 2013–2016.* Edinburgh: Scottish Government. Available from: http://www.gov.scot/Topics/Health/Services/Mental-Health/Dementia/DementiaStrategy1316.

World Health Organisation. (2012) *Dementia: A Public Health Priority.* Geneva, Switzerland: World Health Organization and Alzheimer's Disease International.

Further reading

Dementia care and LGBT communities. (2016) "A good practice paper." Available from: http://www.mhpf.org.uk/sites/default/files/documents/publications/29042016_dementia_care_and_lgbt_communities_a_good_practice_paper.pdf.

NHS Scotland. (2016) "Dementia and equality – meeting the challenge in Scotland." Available from: http://www.healthscotland.scot/media/1226/27797-dementia-and-equality_aug16_english.pdf.

The Mental Health Foundation. (2013) "Losing track of time. Dementia and the ageing prison population: treatment challenges and examples of good practice." Available from: https://www.mentalhealth.org.uk/sites/default/files/losing-track-of-time-2013.pdf.

Watchman, K. (2017) *Intellectual disability and dementia: a guide for families.* London: Jessica Kingsley Publishers.

6 Dementia and the family

Motivations for caring

Janice McAlister and Irene Graham

Introduction

Over the past three decades many government policies and strategic drivers have influenced the change in focus of dementia care from a somewhat arguable institutionalised biomedical model of care to models that are community focused, person-centred and inclusive (Banerjee 2009; Innes and Manthorpe 2013). UK policies in the 1980s and 1990s for example reflected some of this thinking and the expectation that an increased number of older people would require a greater level of care. This was set against a backdrop of an expected reduction in availability of informal carers due in the main to reduction in birth rates, but was also as a result of changes in family structure (Fingerman et al. 2009). The emergence of the "Demographic Time Bomb" and responses to it were founded upon a negative non-productive, dependant image of ageing, with the apparent driver of reducing or transferring to families the expected cost in caring for an ageing population (Knapp et al. 2007). This problem-based view of ageing coincided with a tendency to plan dementia services and models of care from a narrow professional perspective in which family caring existed but was rarely enabled.

More recently many national and international strategic drivers appear to have less of a disease focus and are becoming more person-centred, highlighting the need for people with dementia to be supported to live well within community settings that are both enabling and inclusive (Scottish Government 2010a, 2010b, 2011; WHO 2016, World Alzheimer's Report 2016).

Despite these rising statistics and a plethora of research and academic literature in relation to family caring roles, the level of influence that they have had on social policy appears to be limited (Nolan et al. 2002). There continues to be an expectation of carers adopting the role, with little recognition taken of not only the carers willingness but more importantly their ability to fulfil a caring role (Nolan et al. 1996; Reinhard et al. 2008). Much of the available research and literature surrounding carer experience appears to focus on negative aspects of caring, with a historic trend of highlighting feelings of burden, stress and reduced quality of life, often referred to as Carer Burden (Papastavrou et al. 2007). In contrast to this however many carers voice feelings of positivity around their caring role indicating feelings of satisfaction, fulfilment and improved wellbeing (Mitchell 2001; Ulstein et al. 2007; Reinhard et al. 2008). It has been suggested that there are a range of socio-demographic factors that may impact on carer experience and clinical outcomes, i.e. gender, age, social status and cultural heritage (Bookwala and Schulz 2000; Robinson et al. 2001). Although in contrast to this Nagatomo et al. (1999) found less evidence of a correlation. This chapter will critically discuss carer experience including feelings of stress and caring satisfactions commonly associated with caring for a family member with dementia, with a particular focus on carer profiles, reasons identified for caring and the impact of current strategic drivers. It will be concluded with a summary of findings and the potential impact on clinical practice.

Family structures can be somewhat diverse and complex: for the purpose of this chapter reference to families will encompass both nuclear and extended family members.

Care giver profile

The aetiology and neurodegenerative nature of dementia has been discussed in previous chapters. As a result of this degenerative process there is an expectation of gradual decline and level of functioning, resulting in a possible need for increased level of care and support.

The format of care provision for individuals with dementia is likely to be varied, but there is an increased likelihood that the person will be supported by a network of both informal and formal carers. A high proportion of informal care networks are made up of family and friends with recognition of input from both male and female carers. Current data available from the Office of National Statistics (2013) indicate that caring roles are more likely to be carried out by females than males, with a higher proportion of spouses being identified followed by daughters. The vast majority of carers are aged between 50 and 64 (Brodaty and Donkin 2009; a carer profile which much of the literature suggests is most likely to experience feelings of burden, stress and poor quality of life associated with caring roles (Papastavrou et al. 2007; Banerjee 2014). The reasons for this Etters et al. (2008) suggest are the possibility of a higher proportion of middle age female carers in previous studies, alongside of which, they further indicate that this cohort of carers are more inclined to express their feelings of burden. In contrast to this hypothesis, consideration has to be given to other influencing factors, such as additional family commitments, employment and financial status, pre-morbid relationships and motivation for caring. Within clinical practice, we have found that these multidimensional variables can have a combined impact on carer outcomes. We have frequently encountered individuals with dual caring roles, normally caring for an older parent and younger children, whilst trying to juggle employment commitments or feeling they have to reduce hours of work, which has then financial implications for the family unit. In keeping with the findings of (Kirkman 2011), we would also suggest that within many countries including Scotland there is still evidence of traditional gender roles, with an expectation that female family members will not only adopt but embrace the role of carer.

Box 6.1 Discussion point

Although I wanted to care for my husband and wouldn't have had it any other way. No-one actually asked if this was my choice and how I felt about it. There appeared to be an assumption that I would automatically take on a caring role within our relationship.

Carer's voiceSouth West Scotland

Motivations for caring

People have not forward planned and prepared for their role as a carer for someone with dementia (Contador et al. 2012; Alzheimer's Research UK 2015). The insidious nature of the condition does not lend itself to such forward planning and as such will have a major impact on the life of both the person with dementia and their carer (Fortinsky et al. 2007; Wickson-Griffiths et al. 2014).

Box 6.2 Discussion point

The diagnosis of dementia completely changed the plans we had made for our future. As a couple we had to review our current and future life choices. Although we could still do things together, many things had to be adapted and reshaped.

Carer's voice

The reasons identified by carers for taking on such a life-changing role are varied, from duty, guilt, and responsibility, to reciprocity and love (Brodaty and Donkin 2009; Camden et al. 2011; Quinn et al. 2013). Motives for caring have been identified as major influencing factors on both carer burden and physical ill health, with negative reasons for caring being associated with increased carer burden. Alongside which, pre-disposing factors such as the nature of previous relationships have been noted as having a significant impact (Ablitt et al. 2009); we can hypothesise that a historically poor relationship may have a negative impact on any caring dyad. These are features often encountered, with family members who reluctantly find themselves in a caring role apparently expressing higher levels of emotion. The perceived impact of caring may at times lead to feelings of resentment and anger, particularly in relation to social isolation and financial implications.

In contrast to this however, many carers highlight extremely positive motivational factors for continuing in their caring role, with feelings of satisfaction, pride and companionship being frequently expressed (Wadham et al. 2016).

Box 6.3 Reflective thought

Although there has been a change in the balance of our relationship. We are still a couple and continue to find humour in the strangest and sometimes darkest places. It's important to laugh together.

Carer's voice

Discussion

The impact of the role of carer is multi-faceted and extremely complex with both positive and negative feelings being identified throughout the available literature. It could be argued that neither of these feelings can exist in isolation, and that, as with many relationships, feelings of stress and anxiety may be experienced by carers even in the most positive, satisfying dyad (Ablitt et al. 2009; Braun et al. 2009; Molyneaux 2012).

Box 6.4 Reflective thought

Like any other couple we have good and bad days. We have a normal healthy relationship, we argue and we make up just like everyone else.

Carer's voice

In order to maintain relationship equilibrium, this highlights the importance, need and fundamental right for carers to be seen as equal partners in care, involved in planning and decision making processes. The need for recognition of couple-hood and family as partners forms the basis of recent national and international guidance (WHO 2017).

Taking into account the previously noted carer profile and motivators, it has been suggested that these could ideally be used as predictors of carer stress and as a guide to targeting interventions (Kim et al. 2011). It has also been suggested by Gaugler et al. (2000) in their research into predictors of institutional care, that increased levels of carer burden were a primary catalyst to a long-term care placement being sought. This is in contrast to the findings of Noonan et al. (1996) who found that although carers identified feelings of anxiety and stress it did not pre-empt a relinquishing of their carer role. The positive and negative aspects of caring are not static but tend to be transient and responsive in the main to psychological, physical and environmental factors. From this perspective, it could be argued that through a holistic needs assessment and care planning process, many carers could be better supported in caring for family members with dementia. This idea was conceptualised by Carbonneau et al. (2010) who suggest that interventions which focus and nurture the positive aspects of caring, may have a impact on reducing carer burden and improving the quality of life of both carers and people with dementia.

In relation to research influencing policy, in contrast to Nolan et al. (2002) more recent findings in dementia have had an impact on government policy (Stalker 2003; Carbonneau et al. 2010; Alzheimer's Disease International 2013). This can be seen from documents such as Dementia Standards of Care in Scotland that highlight the need for people with dementia to have carers who are "well supported and educated about dementia". Scotland's Dementia Strategy (Scottish Government 2013) also gave the commitment that people with dementia and their carers receive a year of post diagnostic support. This support framework is based on the 5 and 8 Pillar Models of Care developed by Alzheimer Scotland and is designed to be delivered by an allocated worker. In a further attempt to improve outcomes, this recommendation also became a government HEAT (Health Improvement, Efficiency, Access to Services and Treatment) target for 2013/14 (Scottish Government 2012). Many clinicians are keen to avoid this being viewed as purely a target driven process with the risk of failing to recognise the individual. In the model of delivery of this objective, over the past few years emphasis has been placed on the importance of both carers and people with dementia being seen as individuals with unique needs and as such will require and process information in different formats and at varying rates which are appropriate and tailor made to meet individual needs (Clark et al. 2008; Reinhard et al. 2008). If carer burden is to be reduced and quality of life improved, it is also a priority that post diagnostic support is not viewed in isolation but is part of an individualised holistic care package. If support for carers is to be effective, it should not start at the point of diagnosis, but rather at point of referral to diagnostic services. Effective therapeutic relationships are built up over time, and arguably should start prior to the diagnostic process commencing, a process which can be a major catalyst to stress and distress in both the individual and carers. Effective care management should support the family unit throughout the diagnostic process (Clark et al. 2008).

As was noted previously, there are many factors which can influence the levels of burden and stress experienced by carers. Various government policies have gone some way to reduce these by embracing and driving forward an apparent whole systems qualitative approach to dementia care at national level (Alzheimer's Disease International 2013). This can be evidenced by the introduction of key priorities such as a dementia nurse consultant for each of the NHS Boards in Scotland (Scottish Government 2010b), a role that has a key objective of improving the standard of care for people with dementia and their carers across services. In support of these roles, over 600 people in key positions within health and social service are trained as dementia champions (Scottish Government 2010b, 2013; Banks et al. 2013), who support and work collaboratively in partnership with people with dementia, carers and colleagues across services. In addition to which, staff across, health and social care partnerships, acute care services, voluntary and private sector will receive training within the Promoting Excellence framework (Scottish Government 2011). This framework will ensure the level of staff's skills and knowledge in relation to dementia care is appropriate to their role, enabling them to meet the needs of people with dementia and support and work in partnership with carers.

The need for information and knowledge is also a key component in carer support strategies, with research evidence suggesting that carer education programmes can have a marked influence in improving clinical outcomes for people with dementia and their carers (Brodaty, 1989; Chiverton and Caine 1989). Gormley (2000) further argues that education as a single component has little impact on the reduction of carer burden, and that a multi-dimensional approach is needed. This is a concept that is supported by findings from my own area of clinical practice, where carer education is viewed not as an individual component but part of a holistic care package. There have been times where at the request of carers, education has been facilitated in isolation and on these occasions, we would question the value or impact it has had. We would further suggest that there could be beneficial outcomes in adopting a framework such as Promoting Excellence (Scottish Government 2011) in the development of family carer education programmes.

Conclusion

This chapter has critically discussed the feelings of burden and stress experienced by carers when caring for a family member with dementia. It has highlighted the impact that carer profile and motives for caring may have on carer burden. Although much of the available literature appears to focus on the negative aspects of caring, both the positive and negative feelings associated with caring have been highlighted and whether these can exist in isolation. We have in the main focused on the impact that government policy may have in reducing carer burden and improving clinical outcomes. While there is evidence to suggest that many government recommendations have been initiated at a national level with audit processes incorporated, there is an ongoing need for further research to establish the impact they have had on the lives of people with dementia and their carers.

References

Ablitt, A.J., Jones, G.V. and Muers, J. (2009) "Living with dementia: a systematic review of the influence of relationship factors." *Aging Mental Health*, 13(4): 497–511.

Adams, K.B. (2006) "The transition to care giving: The experience of family members embarking on the dementia caregiving career." *Journal of Gerontology and Social Work*, 47(3–4): 3–29.

Alzheimer's Disease International. (2013) "World Alzheimer Report, Journey of Caring An analysis of long-term care for dementia." London: Alzheimer's Disease International (ADI).

Alzheimer's Research UK. (2015) "Dementia in the Family The impact on carers." Available from: https://www.alzheimersresearchuk.org/wp-content/uploads/2015/12/Dementia-in-the-Family-The-impact-on-carers.pdf.

Andrén, S. and Elmståhl, S. (2007) "Relationships between income, subjective health and caregiver burden in caregivers of people with dementia in group living care: A cross-sectional community-based study." *International Journal of Nursing Studies*, 44(3): 435–446.

Banerjee, S. (2009) *The use of antipsychotic medication for people with dementia: Time for action.* London: Department of Health.

Banerjee, S. (2014) "A flying START for carers of people with dementia." *The Lancet Psychiatry*, 1(7): 489–490.

Banks, P., Waugh, A., Henderson, J., Sharp, B., Brown, M., Oliver, J. and Marland, G. (2013) "Champions Programme in Scotland Enriching the care of patients with dementia in acute settings?" *Dementia*, published online.

Boerner, K., Horowitz, A. and Schlulz, R. (2004) "Positive aspects of caregiving and adaptation to bereavement." *Psychology and Aging*, 19(4): 668–675.

Bookwala, J. and, Schulz, R. (2000) "A comparison of primary stressors, secondary stressors, and depressive symptoms between elderly caregiving husbands and wives: the Caregiver Health Effects Study." *Psychology and Aging*, 15: 607–616.

Braun, M., Scholz, U., Bailey, B., Perren, S., Hornung, R. and Martin, M. (2009) "Dementia caregiving in spousal relationships: A dyadic perspective." *Aging & Mental Health*, 13(3).

Brodaty, H. (1989) "Effect of a training programme to reduce stress in carers of patients with dementia." *BMJ (Clinical Research Ed.)*, 299(6712): 1375.

Brodaty, H. and Donkin, M. (2009) "Family caregivers of people with dementia. Dialogues." *Clinical Neuroscience*, 13(2): 217–228.

Camden, A., Livingston, G. and Cooper, C. (2011) "Reasons why family members become carers and the outcome for the person with dementia: Results from the CARD study." *International Psychogeriatrics*, 23(09): 1442–1450.

Carbonneau, H., Caron, C. and Desrosiers, J. (2010) "Development of a conceptual framework of positive aspects of caregiving in dementia." *Dementia*, August (9): 327–353.

Chiverton, P. and Caine, E. D. (1989) "Education to assist spouses in coping with Alzheimer's disease. A controlled study." *Journal of the American Geriatrics Society*, 37: 593–598.

Clark, C., Chaston, D. and Grant, G. (2008) "Early interventions in dementia: carer led evaluations." In M. Nolan, U. Lundh, G. Gordon and J. Keady. *Partnerships in Family care: Understanding the caregiving career.* Maidenhead, England: Open University Press.

Contador, I., Fernández-Calvo, B., Palenzuela, D.L., Miguéis, S. and Ramos, F. (2012) "Prediction of burden in family caregivers of patients with dementia: a perspective of optimism based on generalized expectancies of control." *Aging Mental Health*, 16: 675–682.

Etters, L., Goodall, D. and Harrison, B.E. (2008) "Caregiver burden among dementia patient caregivers: A review of the literature." *Journal of the American Academy of Nurse Practitioners*, 20(8): 423–428.

Fingerman, K.L., Miller, L. and Seidel, A.J. (2009) "Functions Families Serve in Old Age." In S. H. Qualls and S.H. Zarit (Eds) *Aging Families and Caregiving.* New Jersey: John Wiley. 1–18.

Fortinsky, R.H., Tennen, H., Frank, N. and Affleck, G. (2007) "Health and psychological consequences of caregiving." In C. Aldwin, C. Park and R. Spiro (Eds) *Handbook of health psychology and aging.* New York: Guilford. 227–249.

Gaugler, J.E., Edwards, A.B., Femia, E.E., Zarit, S.H., Stephens, M.P., Townsend, A. and Greene, R. (2000) "Predictors of Institutionalization of Cognitively Impaired Elders: Family Help and the Timing of Placement." *Journal of Gerontology: Psychological Sciences*, 55B(4): 247–255.

Gormley, N. (2000) "The role of dementia training programmes in reducing care-giver burden." *Psychiatric Bulletin*, 24: 41–42.

Innes, A. and Manthorpe, J. (2013) "Developing theoretical understandings of dementia and their application to dementia care policy in the UK." *Dementia*, November 12(6): 682–696.

Kim, H., Chang, M., Rose, K. and Kim, S. (2011) "Predictors of caregiver burden in caregivers of individuals with dementia." *Journal of Advance Nursing*, 68(4): 846–855.

Kirkman, A. (2011) "Caring 'from duty and the heart': Gendered work and Alzheimer's disease." *Women's Studies Journal*, 25(1).

McDonnell, E. and Ryan, A.A. (2013) "The experience of sons caring for a parent with dementia." *Dementia*, 13(6): 788–802.

Mitchell, E. (2001) "Managing carer stress: An evaluation of a stress management programme for carers of people with dementia." *British Journal of Occupational Therapy*, 63(4): 179–184.

Molyneaux, V. J., Butchard, S., Simpson, J. and Murray, C. (2012) "The co-construction of couplehood in dementia." *Dementia: The International Journal of Social Research and Practice*, 11: 483–502.

Nagatomo, I., Akasaki, Y., Uchida, M., Tominaga, M., Hashiguchi, W. and Takigawa, M. (1999) "Gender of demented patients and specific family relationship of caregiver to patients influence mental fatigue and burdens on relatives as caregivers." *International Journal of Geriatric Psychiatry*, 14: 618–625.

Nolan, M.R., Grant, G. and Keady, J. (1996) *Understanding Family Care: A Multidimensional Model of Caring and Coping.* Buckingham: Open University Press.

Nolan, M., Ryan, T., Enderby, P. and Reid, D. (2002) "Towards a more inclusive vision of dementia care practice and research." *Dementia*, 1(2): 193–211.

Noonan, A., Tennstedt, S. and Rebelsky, F. (1996) "Making the Best of It: Themes of Meaning among Informal Caregivers to the Elderly." *Journal of Aging Studies*, 10(4): 313–327.

Office of National Statistics (2013) "Full story: The gender gap in unpaid care provision: is there an impact on health and economic position." Available from: http://www.ons.gov.uk/ons/dcp171776_310295.pdf (accessed 04/03/2014).

Papastavrou, E., Kalokerinou, A., Papacostas, S.S., Tsangari, H. and Sourtzi, P. (2007) "Caring for a relative with dementia: Family caregiver burden." *Journal of Advanced Nursing*, 58(5): 446–457.

Quinn, C., Clare, L. and Woods, R.T. (2013) "Balancing needs: The role of motivations, meanings and relationship dynamics in the experience of informal caregivers of people with dementia." *Sage*, 14(2): 220–237.

Reinhard, S., Given, B., Huhtala, N. and Bemis, A. (2008) "Supporting Family Caregivers." In Hughes, R.G. (Ed) *Providing Care in Patient Safety and Quality: An Evidence-Based Handbook for Nurses*, Rockville: Agency for Healthcare Research and Quality (US).

Robinson, K., Adkisson, P. and Weinrich, S. (2001) "Problem behaviour, caregiver reactions, and impact among caregivers of persons with Alzheimer's disease." *Journal of Advanced Nursing* 36: 573–582.

Robinson, J., Fortinsky, R., Kleppinger, A., Shugrue, N. and Porter, M. (2009) "A broader view of family caregiving: effects of caregiving and caregiver conditions on depressive symptoms, health, work, and social isolation." *Journal of Gerontology: Social Sciences*, 64B (6): 788–798.

Scottish Government. (2010a) "Caring Together: The Carers Strategy for Scotland 2010–2015." Edinburgh: Scottish Government.

Scottish Government. (2010b) "Scotland's National Dementia Strategy." Edinburgh: Scottish Government.

Scottish Government. (2011) "Promoting Excellence: A framework for all health and social services staff working with people with dementia, their families and carer." Edinburgh: Scottish Government.

Scottish Government. (2012) "NHS Scotland Local Delivery Plan Guidance 2013/14." Edinburgh: Scottish Government.

Scottish Government. (2013) "Scotland's National Dementia Strategy, From Promise to Practice." Edinburgh: Scottish Government.

Spillman, B.C. and Long, S.K. (2009) "Does high caregiver stress predict nursing home entry?" *Inquiry*, 46(2): 140–161.

Stalker, K. (2003) *Reconceptualising Work with Carers new Directions for Policy and Practice.* London and Philadelphia: Jessica Kingsley Publishers.

Ulstein, I., Bruun, Wyller T. and Engedal, K. (2007) "The relative stress scale, a useful instrument to identify various aspects of carer burden in dementia?" *International Journal of Geriatric Psychiatry*, 22(1): 61–67.

Wadham, O., Simpson, J., Rust, J. and Murray, C. (2016) "Couples' shared experiences of dementia: a meta-synthesis of the impact upon relationships and couplehood." *Aging & Mental Health*, 20(5).

WHO. (2016) "Draft Global Action Plan on the Public Health Response to Dementia 2017–2025." Available from: http://apps.who.int/gb/ebwha/pdf_files/EB140/B140_28-en.pdf?ua=1.

Wickson-Griffiths, A., Kaasalainen, S., Ploeg, J. and McAiney, C. (2014) "A Review of Advance Care Planning Programs in Long-Term Care Homes: Are They Dementia Friendly?" *Nursing Research and Practice*, Article ID 875897. doi:10.1155/2014/875897.

World Alzheimer's Report. (2016) "Improving healthcare for people living with dementia: Coverage, quality and costs now and in the future." Available from: https://www.alz.co.uk/research/WorldAlzheimerReport2016.pdf.

7 Dementia-friendly communities

Sandra Shafii and Arlene Crockett

Introduction

21st-century health and social care strategy in Scotland coalesces around an agenda characterised by person-centredness, a focus on personal outcomes, supporting people to remain in their own homes safely and confidently for as long as possible, building on the assets of people and communities and supporting people to take more control of their health and wellbeing and their care arrangements.

A recognition that formal health and social care services could not continue to meet demand and fulfil strategic and policy direction in traditional configurations led to the integration of Scotland's health and social care services in 2016 (Scottish Government 2016).

Alongside this changing health and care landscape is the acknowledgement that dementia poses one of the most important health and social challenges to our society now and in the future (Alzheimer's Disease International 2013) This acknowledgment has led to a focus on how people living with dementia within this landscape can be enabled to live an ordinary everyday life, feel valued and contribute as full citizens in society.

If people are to seek help at an early stage in their dementia journey, make decisions about how they wish their future care to be organised and thereafter to live well with dementia within their chosen communities, individuals and local communities need to understand the disease and know how they can make a difference to those living with dementia.

This can only be achieved by raising awareness of dementia, challenging stigma, supporting communities to understand the impact of the disease on the lives of those living with dementia and developing ways in which everyone can react positively and offer support to their fellow citizens.

The "dementia-friendly community" social movement has emerged as one response to these challenges and is gaining momentum in Scotland, the wider United Kingdom and across the world.

Whilst there are many definitions of a "dementia-friendly community", Alzheimer's Disease International – The Global Voice on Dementia – defines a dementia-friendly community as:

"a place or culture in which people with dementia and their carers are empowered, supported and included in society, understand their rights and recognise their full potential" (Alzheimer's Disease International 2013).

The importance of the concept of dementia-friendly communities fits with the needs of our human rights and disability rights to be recognised. In the same way as any other person with a disability, we should be supported to remain independent in our communities for as long as possible.

Kate Swaffer, Dementia Alliance International (Alzheimer's Disease International 2018)

In 2012, the Prime Minister of the United Kingdom set a challenge to deliver major improvements in dementia care and research. One of the three champion groups set up in response to this challenge had a focus on the creation of dementia-friendly communities.

A component of this UK group's work was working in partnership with the Dementia Action Alliance to develop evidence on what a dementia-friendly community is. The Alzheimer's Society and British Standards Institute subsequently produced PAS1365 – a Code of Practice for Dementia-Friendly Communities (The British Standards Institution 2015). This PAS (Publicly Available Specification) was launched on 9 July 2015.

Scotland's approach to developing dementia-friendly communities

The Charter of Rights for People with Dementia and Their Carers in Scotland (Cross Party Group on Alzheimer's 2009) was a landmark publication for dementia care and treatment in Scotland and beyond. The Charter gave strategic importance to a human rights based approach to the development of policy and practice.

> People with dementia and their carers (family members and friends) have the same human rights as every other citizen. However, it is widely recognised that, in addition to the impact of the illness, they face cultural, social and economic barriers to fulfilling these rights. This charter aims to empower people with dementia, those who support them and the community as a whole, to ensure their rights are recognised and respected.

In pursuance of the Human Rights Act 1998 and The Scotland Act 1998, a key principle of the Charter of Rights was that people living with dementia enjoyed "full and effective participation and inclusion in society", thereby challenging stigma and discrimination and bringing dementia and citizenship into sharp focus.

In March 2016, Scotland's emerging National Dementia Strategy (2017–2020) (Scottish Government 2017) proposed to continue to maintain its focus on this human rights based approach including support to "local strategic approaches to promote and complement bottom-up, community-led Dementia-Friendly Community initiatives and utilize these assets as part of service- and support- redesign".

Including the development of dementia-friendly communities explicitly within a national dementia strategy and stating the role that they play, endorses the relevance of dementia-friendly communities in an overarching framework of good dementia care and further endorsed the direction that Scotland had so far taken in developing its approach to this social movement.

Scotland's approach had been developing organically since the first Dementia-Friendly Town Centre initiative launched in September 2012 in Motherwell, North Lanarkshire.

The Motherwell experience

Motherwell Town Centre Dementia-Friendly Community had its beginnings in 2011 as part of a development driven by North Lanarkshire's status as a national Dementia Demonstrator Site.

The process: designing Motherwell Dementia-Friendly Town Centre

As an initial step to implementing Scotland's National Dementia Strategy 2010–2013, conversations had taken place in North Lanarkshire with people living with dementia, their families and carers about "who, what and where" mattered to them when living with dementia in their community.

A range of partnerships events involving people living with dementia, families, carers and representatives from the public and third sector groups were held to hear the voice of lived experience. Appreciative Inquiry was the evidence-based tool used during the consultation stage to create a vision of the desired change.

The Appreciative Inquiry model engaged everyone in discussions and ensured that stories grounded in real experience were gathered and heard. These conversations focussed on the positive aspects of people's lives, what worked well and what needed to happen to leverage that collective positivity to help grow the kind of community people wanted to live within.

During the inquiry process, people living with dementia in North Lanarkshire identified shops, supermarkets, businesses, banks, post offices, libraries, transport services, faith groups and social and recreational groups as being of importance to them in living an ordinary everyday life.

They also identified community health services such as general practice, opticians and dentists as being key to staying well – a crucial factor in supporting them to remain in their own homes.

They spoke about self-efficacy, feeling valued as citizens and the importance of feeling safe and secure within their homes and wider communities. Feeling in control of their lives, contributing to their communities and staying connected to family and friends were central to feeling that they were living life to the full.

Box 7.1 Discussion point

What matters to me? (Laughs) I matter to me! Me and my wee life in my own wee house… that's what matters to me. I don't want anything special just because I have dementia. I just want to live my life with my friends and family. Life is what you make it you know!

Betty, North Lanarkshire 2011

The responses to the inquiry questions were gathered and analysed. Resonance was found with the domains of instruments based on empirical research that measure "quality of life" (such as WHOQOL-100 and QOL-AD) or give an overarching framework for the measurement of health and wellbeing including mental health (such as Eurostat 8 + 1 Dimensions of Quality of Life and WEMWBS). The visions of living life with dementia were mapped with the quality of life, process and change outcomes described in Talking Point's evidence based personal outcomes approach.

The responses to the questions were then used to build a framework on which to take forward the development of a dementia-friendly community in Motherwell Town Centre.

A partnership working group was formed from health and social care and the third sector with the task of developing and testing a dementia-friendly community model which had practicality and sustainability as key components. The first stage was to reach a definition of what was meant by being "dementia friendly". Alzheimer Scotland subsequently further developed the working definition from Motherwell and now uses the following description of a dementia-friendly community:

> A dementia-friendly community is made up of the whole community – shop assistants, public service workers, faith groups, businesses, police, fire and ambulance staff, bus drivers, school pupils, clubs and societies and community leaders – people who are committed to working together and helping people with dementia to remain a part of their community and not become apart from it. This involves learning a little about dementia and doing very simple and practical things that can make an enormous difference to people living with the condition.
>
> (Alzheimer Scotland 2016)

Motherwell Town Centre area was chosen as the target "community" as it had a wide range of the shops, businesses, services and organisations, faith communities and forms of transport that people had said was important to them.

Embedding the dementia-friendly community work within a customer care approach was the means of engagement with the target businesses and organisations. Logos, straplines, marketing and information materials, "Hints and Tips", flyers and resources were developed in line with Alzheimer Scotland branding to give the developing model an identity and set it within a policy context and wider strategic direction.

The straplines developed by the initiative, "Dementia is Everyone's Business", "Everyone Knows Someone with Dementia" and "This is about me and mine and you and yours" opened not just the doors to shops and businesses but also opened the hearts and minds of everyone who engaged in the work.

The community response to the dementia-friendly community initiative was enthusiastic, unequivocal and practical. During conversations with businesses and shops, personal stories of living with dementia were shared and commitments to support people living with dementia were made. Conversations with those shops and businesses raised awareness of dementia, its impact on people, families and carers, the importance of citizenship and maintenance of personal, social and community connections. Shops and businesses that signed up were also able to see how being part of a dementia-friendly community programme would say something important about their value base, bring benefits in reputation and help fulfil corporate social responsibility obligations.

Businesses and organisations made commitments. At a minimum, these commitments included ensuring that their staff received "Hints and Tips" on how to support someone with dementia if they came into their workplace and how to treat them with dignity and respect.

However, more than simply giving information about dementia, the dementia-friendly community initiative worked with businesses and organisations to develop action plans.

These action plans led to mutually beneficial relationships. New partnerships with shops and businesses in the community were made, assets identified, shared benefits such as reciprocal training opportunities were realised and offers of help and support with knowledge, skills, resources and premises emerged.

Awareness training was made available to the businesses and organisations. Training covered topics such as understanding dementia, the impact of the environment and dementia-friendly signage.

The Motherwell Dementia-Friendly Town Centre initiative proved to be successful. It captured imagination and attracted media attention locally, nationally and internationally. The simple methodology and tool kit of resources developed were made publicly available on Alzheimer Scotland's website.

Links were made with other UK and European countries who were also developing dementia-friendly community approaches and methodologies. Learning and resources were shared and "Hints and Tips" was translated into other languages.

The initiative's success was based firmly on the strong foundation of that initial step – listening to the voices of those living with dementia in the North Lanarkshire community and hearing about what was important to them and about their hopes and aspirations for their future within their community.

Learning from Motherwell

Motherwell's dementia-friendly community initiative was set clearly within the policy and strategy direction for health and social care and dementia care in Scotland. However, developing and working towards a dementia-friendly community takes time, effort, commitment, energy, openness, sharing of assets and the support of all sectors in society.

If dementia-friendly communities are to play their part in an overarching framework of good dementia care, then they need to be given status within a public health and social care context and viewed as an essential component in building the community capacity and resilience required to meet the challenges facing health and social care in the future.

Key learning from the Motherwell experience can be grouped under the following headings: definition, people, planning, partnership, places and performance.

Definition

Developing a local definition was felt to be important as building the dementia-friendly community model in Motherwell depended upon community led co-production and had to correspond to the vision created by local people living with dementia.

The Motherwell experience supports the view that agreeing that definition right at the beginning of the process is critical to success and is the essential first stage from which ownership emerges and actions flow.

There are several definitions emerging from practice across the globe such as the one offered by ADI and from elsewhere in the UK (PAS1365) and Europe.

> **Box 7.2 Learning point**
>
> Dementia-friendly communities are geographic areas where people with dementia are understood, respected and supported, and confident they can contribute to community life. In a dementia-friendly community people are aware of and understand dementia, and people with dementia feel included and involved, and have choice and control over their day-to-day lives. A dementia-friendly community is

made up of individuals, businesses, organizations, services, and faith communities that support the needs of people with dementia.

(PAS 1365)

People

Developing a dementia-friendly community begins with people.

Listening to the experiences of those living with dementia, hearing their stories and having positive appreciative conversations about life in their communities creates definition and direction.

Hearing from the wider community and community leaders about the issues and challenges around day to day life gave helpful background to developing priorities, understanding the community context, identification of assets and introductions to people who could help with the work.

Motherwell's project team drew on a range of skills and abilities – from people with vision, to people with practical skills and those who liked attention to detail. The team reflected the assets based approach underpinning Motherwell's dementia-friendly community model. The members of the team were asked to acknowledge, share and contribute personal skills, talents, abilities and attributes to the work as well as being representative of their organisations.

Experience showed that people involved in developing dementia-friendly communities need to be committed to the concept. They need to be warm, engaging, friendly, flexible and enthusiastic. Good communication skills, ability to talk to a range of people from differing and diverse backgrounds and experiences, they need to understand and be fluent with the key messages underpinning the work and good negotiation skills were all essential qualities of the team members.

Planning

Starting with the definition of what is meant by "community" is essential. A community can be anything from a city to a town to a village; from a geographical area such as a county to a single street or town centre; from a shopping mall to a care home.

Researching and gathering data from a wide variety of sources will build a real-time picture of that community.

Data could include information about population, deprivation indicators, community hot spots and social issues. Identifying assets such as buildings, places, community leaders and activists and any planned or developing projects that might link to the development of a dementia-friendly community can further shape and inform the dementia-friendly community design.

Access to expertise around asset-based approaches to community development and community capacity building can be helpful in supporting dementia-friendly community planning.

Having knowledge of local planning projects is useful as this may present an opportunity to influence future plans and include dementia-friendly environmental elements at design or planning stages.

Exploring the defined dementia-friendly community area through the lens of those with lived experience of dementia and using what people living with dementia said about who, what and where was important to them will target resources, define priorities and progress the dementia-friendly community plan.

It will also build a picture of the partnerships needed to shape the dementia-friendly community design.

Partnerships

> **Box 7.3 Discussion point**
>
> 43 Part of the response to the challenges is about effective partnership working between the NHS, local government and the voluntary and private sectors, respecting the separate contribution and capability of each, but also understanding our collective ability to achieve change through integrated working.
>   Scotland's National Dementia Strategy 2010–2013 (Scottish Government 2010)

The Motherwell initiative was built on partnerships founded on the concept of "shareholding" as opposed to the more familiar term of "stakeholding". The concept of shareholding was fundamental to the Motherwell dementia-friendly community process as it brought a fresh sense of shared investment and ownership in the dementia-friendly community and its aspirations. Using the term "shareholder" initiated new conversations about involvement, equality and relationship within the partnership.

Responsibility and accountability for the development of the dementia-friendly community was owned and shared by the partnership working group. Fundamental to the process was the agreement that no one organisation or group could assume leadership for the process or should be the natural lead agency.

Places

Conversations with people living with dementia identified the places that mattered to them and the responses from these conversations identified a range of built and natural environments, local community assets and resources. These places were then targeted in the first phase of Motherwell's initiative.

The design and physical attributes of built and natural environments contribute to the context of a dementia-friendly community and can influence the physical, emotional and psychological wellbeing of all citizens.

The Motherwell initiative made links with the Memory Friendly Neighbourhood collaboration between research centres at the Universities of Stirling and Edinburgh. This programme recognises the "policy prominent concept of dementia-friendly communities" and "meets the urgent need for insights to guide the development of environments for ageing-in-place and lifelong social inclusion for those affected by dementia".

Performance

The Motherwell Dementia-Friendly Town Centre initiative is an example of "learning by doing".

The foundation for the initiative was based within policy and strategy and rooted in the concepts of social inclusion, co-creation, co-production and true partnership working across all three elements of society – the public, private and third sector.

Reflection and evaluation of the work was a key component of being a part of a national Dementia Demonstrator Site and the initiative used a range of methods to gather information about the difference the dementia-friendly community approach was making to the experience of those living with dementia.

The basic focus of the initiative was on good customer care and therefore the "mystery shopper" approach was used.

Test phone calls were also made to businesses and organisations that had signed up to become dementia-friendly. People were asked a range of questions and their responses were gathered and analysed.

Numbers of staff receiving "Hints and Tips" and undertaking training were collected, and environmental audits were undertaken.

Motherwell Dementia-Friendly Town Centre gained recognition in Scotland, the UK and internationally winning several awards Invitations to share learning and to present at national and international events were received. Further recognition came from European Foundation's Initiative on Dementia (EFID) in 2014 when North Lanarkshire was awarded funds to support further local dementia-friendly community development within its culturally and linguistically diverse communities.

Learning from Motherwell's Mosque and Muslim Community Project 2014–2015

The Dementia-Friendly Community work in Motherwell demonstrated that the Black and Minority Ethnic (BME) Community was under-represented in existing services and highlighted an inequality of access and knowledge about dementia and dementia services within this group. In March 2014, an award of 10,000 Euros was received from the European Foundations Initiative in Dementia to develop a dementia-friendly community response to the local BME community in North Lanarkshire.

2011 census data as well as discussions with partners in third sector groups demonstrated that the most prominent community in North Lanarkshire was the Pakistani/Muslim Community. The project worker and partners from the local Carers Trust pooled their resources and developed an extension to the reach of existing support in North Lanarkshire for BME communities and faith communities.

Box 7.4 Discussion point

Muslims are not only in the Mosque. Go into the communities to support them. They will come.

Lanarkshire Mosque and Muslim Community project 2014

The Muslim community acknowledge that they need to work to reduce stigma around dementia. They recognise that raising awareness of dementia and talking about the disease will support future generations of women who are traditional carers within their families.

Findings from the project showed that years of marginalisation of the Muslim group in society means there is still a lot to of work to do with service planners and providers to build trust and break down barriers.

The Lanarkshire Mosque and Muslim Community project started a movement for change and a sense of ownership within the BME community. This community are now open to working in partnership with Alzheimer Scotland and other partners to make a difference for the future.

Learning from this project contributed to the development of Commitment 16 of Scotland's National Dementia Strategy 2013–2016 (Scottish Government 2013) which began to address equality issues. The project also demonstrated the importance of cultural competency when developing dementia-friendly communities and working with culturally and linguistically diverse communities. Cultural competency can be defined as the ability of an individual, organisation or practitioner to recognise the cultural beliefs, attitudes and health practices of diverse populations and to apply that knowledge in every intention; at the systems level or at the individual level, to produce a positive health outcome.

Moving forward

Since Motherwell's dementia-friendly town centre launch (2012), Scotland has taken up the UK dementia-friendly communities and Dementia Friends challenges. The Dementia Friends Scotland programme commenced in 2014 and Scotland has assimilated this initiative into its dementia-friendly community developments.

Scotland's commitment to the dementia-friendly community movement was given further weight in April 2015 when the Life Changes Trust invested £3.4 million over a period of three years in 14 dementia-friendly communities across Scotland. The communities that received the investment are diverse; ranging from "communities of interest" to specific geographical areas or towns to reflect the reality of people's everyday lives.

There are several examples of dementia-friendly community initiatives in Scotland to explore – from East Sutherland to Dementia-Friendly Prestwick, to city-wide approaches as in Glasgow, Edinburgh and Stirling to areas reflecting Scotland's more rural and township communities as in Portobello, Dumfries and Galloway, West Dunbartonshire and South Lanarkshire.

Each of these communities has taken the dementia-friendly community concept and shaped their response consistent with their own circumstances, hopes and aspirations building on who, what and where matters to their citizens who are living with dementia.

Evaluations from York and Bradford dementia-friendly communities (Dean et al. 2015) echo the Motherwell experience and give weight to the need for a national strategic commitment to underpin development. In Bradford, people raised the issue of a rights campaign which would challenge "decision makers, legislators and funders" to move the creation of dementia-friendly communities from a paper based commitment into mainstream with accompanying investment to support dementia-friendly community development. York's dementia-friendly community evaluation findings suggested that although there is a strategic commitment to dementia-friendly communities they did not find widespread evidence of delivery. The concept of basing the movement on a rights basis was also explored in York's evaluation (Dean et al. 2015).

> The relationship between the concept of a dementia-friendly community and a 'rights movement' is interesting. For some a dementia-friendly community is about making a place easier to live in for a person with dementia, for others the notion of inclusion is more explicitly about rights.

Importantly the evidence base for dementia-friendly communities is still building. Experiences and learning are being shared and basic guidelines and principles are emerging.

As a global social movement, the dementia-friendly community is gaining traction.

Scotland's strategic commitments based on a "bottom-up community-led basis" (Scottish Government Scotland's National Dementia Strategy 2017–2020) supports an organic approach to local development, welcoming diversity in dementia-friendly community design. Interestingly the Scottish approach also reflects the uniqueness of the dementia experience for the individual.

Box 7.5 The cornerstones of a dementia-friendly community

In addressing the twin objectives of reducing stigma and increasing understanding of dementia and empowering people with dementia, Alzheimer's Disease International suggests that the four essential elements needed to support a dementia-friendly community are people, communities, organisations and partnerships.

Alzheimer's Disease International (2016)

References

Alzheimer Scotland. (2016) "Dementia Friendly Communities." Available from: https://www.alzscot.org/dementia_friendly_communities.

Alzheimer's Disease International. (2013) "World Alzheimer Report 2013. Journey of Caring – An analysis of long-term care for dementia – Executive Summary." Available from https://www.alz.co.uk/research/WorldAlzheimerReport2013ExecutiveSummary.pdf.

Alzheimer's Disease International. (2016a) "Principles of a Dementia Friendly Community." Available from: https://www.alz.co.uk/dementia-friendly-communities/principles.

Alzheimer's Disease International. (2016b) "Dementia Friendly Communities." Available from: https://www.alz.co.uk/dementia-friendly-communities.

Cross Party Group on Alzheimer's. (2009) "Charter of Rights for People with Dementia and their Carers in Scotland." Available from: https://www.alzscot.org/assets/0000/2678/Charter_of_Rights.pdf.

Dean, J., Silversides, K., Crampton, J. and Wrigley, J. (2015) "Evaluation of the Bradford Dementia Friendly Communities Programme. Joseph Rowntree Foundation." Available from: https://www.jrf.org.uk/report/evaluation-bradford-dementia-friendly-communities-programme.

Scottish Government. (2010) "Scotland's National Dementia Strategy 2010–2013." Available from: http://www.gov.scot/Resource/Doc/324377/0104420.pdf.

Scottish Government. (2013) "Scotland's National Dementia Strategy 2013–2016." Available from: http://www.gov.scot/Resource/0042/00423472.pdf.

Scottish Government. (2016) "Health and Social Care Delivery Plan." Available from http://www.gov.scot/Resource/0051/00511950.pdf.

Scottish Government. (2017) "Scotland's National Dementia Strategy 2017–2020." Available from: http://www.gov.scot/Resource/0052/00521773.pdf.

The British Standards Institution. (2015) "Code of practice for the recognition of dementia-friendly communities in England BSI Standards Limited 2015." Available from: https://www.housinglin.org.uk/_assets/Resources/Housing/OtherOrganisation/BSI_Dementia_friendly.pdf.

Useful websites

Alzheimer's Disease International: https://www.alz.co.uk/dementia-friendly-communities.

Alzheimer's Society: https://www.alzheimers.org.uk/info/20079/dementia_friendly_communities.

Alzheimer Scotland: http://www.alzscot.org/dementia_friendly_communities.

Joseph Rowntree Foundation: https://www.jrf.org.uk/people/dementia.

Life Changes Trust: https://www.lifechangestrust.org.uk/projects/dementia-friendly-communities.

Memory Friendly Neighbourhoods: http://memoryfriendly.org.uk/.

8   The care environment and dementia

Mary Marshall

It is impossible in a short chapter, to cover the whole field of designing for dementia. Fundamentally it is about compensating for the impairments of old age as well as dementia. This chapter uses five people with dementia, each in different circumstances, to illustrate how some design features can make a huge difference to their functioning, safety and well-being. **Design is a seriously neglected non-pharmaceutical intervention.** The aim of this chapter is simply to raise awareness and interest in this key intervention.

Mrs Hawkins lived most of her life in a small flat, furnished mainly when she got married 50 years ago. Over the years she and her husband had replaced worn out items but the basic furniture was from the 1950s. She inherited some ornaments when her mother died, which had great meaning for her although her daughter thought they were hideous. When she went into a care home with a dementia unit last year, her daughter bought her a lot of new things including new ornaments. The only items that went with her from home were photographs of her wedding, children and grandchildren. Mrs Hawkins was utterly bewildered and is still totally perplexed about where she is. No amount of people telling her the bedroom was now her home made sense to her.

It is easy for staff and relatives to fail to see the importance of the environment – from the whole building down to the tiny details of ornaments and pictures. People quite rightly focus on relationships and care that are absolutely crucial. But the environment is the context in which this happens. In this chapter I want to explain the extent to which the environment is a major non-pharmaceutical intervention for people with dementia and conversely, the extent to which it can cause unnecessary disability. I also want to look at the way that a therapeutic environment makes things *possible* for staff and people with dementia; although of course it does not make things happen. I will focus on the transition from home to a care home, day care or hospital, since this is very often a problem for people whose ability to adapt and understand is impaired by their dementia. I will also look at people with different levels of impairment. I will try to achieve these aims by means of stories of people with dementia moving into new places. Key lessons will be highlighted.

Putting yourself in the shoes of someone like Mrs Hawkins is the best place to start. She had the symptoms of dementia for ten years. When she was diagnosed eight years ago, she initially had some understanding of her diagnosis. She was able to continue to cope at home since it was very familiar. She had familiar routines, her neighbours kept an eye on her and her daughter did her shopping and spent a lot of time at weekends cleaning the house and making sure her mother was coping. Mrs Hawkins then had a fall and was admitted to hospital where she deteriorated sharply in both her mobility and her competence. She was clearly not going to be able to live alone. To try and help her understand this, she went home for a weekend and left home for the last time on the following Monday.

When she was admitted to the care home, Mrs Hawkins needed a place that was understandable, safe and where she could continue her routines as far as possible. To make it understandable, her bedroom should have been full of familiar items, so that she was able to appreciate that this was her space. Although the room was pleasantly furnished by the owner, it should have had furniture, carpet and curtains that made sense to someone whose taste was formed in the 1950s.

Box 8.1 Key point: Low cost

- Bedrooms should be familiar with as many meaningful belongings in as possible (even if some relatives for the best of reasons want to buy new things)
- Staff may need to explain this to the relatives

Mrs Hawkins had perceptual as well as cognitive impairments. Her brain was failing to interpret what she was seeing and this meant that she was inclined to "see" a change in the tone of the floor as a step, to see frightening things in patterns and to see specks as litter. This is not uncommon in people with Alzheimer's disease.

Box 8.2 Learning point

Agnes Houston who has Alzheimer's disease and perceptual impairments says in her DVD and booklet: "I call it brain blindness which means your eyes see, but your brain doesn't interpret the information immediately".

Unfortunately Mrs Hawkins's bedroom floor was a light wood effect vinyl that contrasted strongly with the darker carpet in the corridor which meant that she thought she had to step downwards into her bedroom. There was also a silver strip along the threshold and another along the threshold into the en-suite. Both made Mrs Hawkins anxious. A falls risk was added to her environment by ill-considered flooring.

Box 8.3 Key points:

- Be aware of perceptual as well as cognitive impairments
- Avoid flooring contrast of more than 5 LRV, specks, wavy lines in wallpaper and fabrics, strong patterns

(LRV is the way tone is measured. It means Light Reflectance Value. It goes from 0–100. 0 is black (no reflection) and 100 is white (maximum reflection). All paint samples and tins will have the LRV on them, and any interior designer or architect can advise.)

On leaving her bedroom, Mrs Hawkins entered a corridor with a corner at each end. She had no idea which way to go (see Marquardt 2011 on wayfinding). She needed a directional sign pointing to the communal areas. Directly opposite was another room with an identical door. Mrs Hawkins frequently crossed the corridor and went into this room. Staff had to help her to walk to the lounge because she could not find her way on her own, although she was able to walk the distance with her walker. They also had to help her find her room on her return. She failed to understand the number, name and photograph of herself. This is unnecessary disability related to poor design.

Box 8.4 Key points: Low cost

- Most people with dementia need to be able to see where they want to go. They usually have neither the memory, nor the ability to learn where places are. If this is not possible, a clear sign can help
- Doors should be made recognisable by items that are meaningful to the person. This will be different for different people. A memory box would not have made sense to Mrs Hawkins but the number of her own home on the door would have helped her find it

---

Box 8.5 Key points:

- Bedroom doors should not face each other
- Clear signage can be very useful (see also Mrs Patel below). Signs should be mounted 1.2 metres from the floor

---

Having got to the lounge, Mrs Hawkins immediately understood its function with its comfortable chairs and domestic furniture. The chairs contrasted with the floor and walls as did the small tables, which made them highly visible. The lounge/dining area was open plan which was a great help to Mrs Hawkins who could see and understand the dining area because it had small tables and dining chairs. It also had a counter kitchen along the side so Mrs Hawkins could see a sink, taps and a kettle. This was very reassuring to her and she coped well with understanding mealtimes and was able to help lay the tables and clear them afterwards. However she was not eating well. It took staff several weeks to work out why not. The reason was inadequate lighting. Dining room lighting should be 300 lux at the tables and any serving areas if people are to see their food properly. Staff were well aware of the need for food to contrast with the plates and for the plates to contrast with the table so this was not a problem. Improving the lighting helped both Mrs Hawkins and some of her fellow residents.

In the lounge/dining room Mrs Hawkins thought she was in a club and she was comfortable, but she had no understanding at all that she could not then go home since her bedroom was in no sense her "home". She was constantly asking when she was going home which was very upsetting to her and to the staff.

Box 8.6 Key point: Low cost

- Significant contrast in tone is essential for the ageing eye to see things like furniture, plates, food etc. This means a difference of over 30 LRV (Fuggle 2013)

Box 8.7 Key points

- Twice the normal levels of light are needed for the ageing eye. Take care that there is no glare which is painful for the ageing eye
- Open plan is really helpful as are appropriate furniture and fittings. Avoid clutter which can be distracting and confusing
- Activities can be more likely if possibilities, such as a kitchenette or shed, are part of the design

Mr Calder was admitted to an acute mental health unit for assessment because he was becoming very aggressive to his wife. She had coped with his dementia for some years though it had not been easy. He had been a steel worker and increasingly wanted to go out to work, getting very angry when he was prevented. If she allowed him to go out, he got lost very quickly and on several occasions he was brought back by police. When he threatened violence to a visiting social worker, he was admitted under section.

Mr Calder did not thrive in the unit. He was a reasonably fit man, although 82, and he walked up and down the main corridor all day often frightening other patients and their visitors. He was constantly trying to leave the unit through the front door, which was very obvious because all ward traffic came and went through it. He shared a bedroom bay with three other people. It had a shared toilet which he rarely found without help. There was a staff hand washing sink in the bay and he usually urinated in this. He was very particular about cleanliness and looked for a sink to wash his hands without success. If he found the en-suite, he could not understand the tap and often became very angry and upset. He found the dining room particularly stressful and often shouted and refused to eat.

If the staff had been able to assess and change the environment, they would have wanted to change it in many ways. They would have liked to make the front door a lot less conspicuous and to direct attention to other rooms. Clearly they could not provide single rooms, although there are numerous studies showing that single rooms are better for people with dementia (e.g. Wilkes et al. 2005). This single room could have had a toilet visible from the bed to enable him to find it quickly. It would have had cross-head taps clearly labelled hot and cold. They would have liked to enable Mr Calder to "go out to work". He, like many active men who have done physical work all their lives, needed somewhere to go which made sense to him. An activities room with bits of machinery would have been a huge bonus. They would also have liked to make the outside area easier to supervise so that Mr Calder could have walked off some of his energy in the fresh air. The "workshop" could usefully have been outside to enhance the impression of going out to work. They would certainly have liked to make the dining room less noisy. For reasons of infection control, there were no sound absorbent surfaces at all in the dining room, which as a result, reverberated strongly at mealtimes – giving the staff headaches let alone the patients. Acoustic panels, perhaps designed to look like an attractive art panel, could have soaked up some of the reverberation. Mr Calder, already an angry and frustrated man, was made worse by an environment that felt hostile to him.

Box 8.8 Key points: Low cost

- Conceal the front door by painting it the same colour as adjoining walls and ensuring there is attractive activity elsewhere
- Reduce noise – perhaps the major cause of distressed behaviour for anyone with dementia. Noise is unwanted sound, and it is even more problematic when the person feels powerless to do anything about it

---

Box 8.9 Key points:

- Single rooms
- Easily accessible and visible toilet with understandable taps, flush and shower controls
- Design for activities appropriate to the users
- Easily observed, accessible, safe outside space

Mrs Patel's daughter-in-law was struggling to cope. Mrs Patel senior was bored and demanding, which made looking after her husband and two grown up children really difficult. Mrs Patel junior needed to shop, clean, cook and do all her other housework, which was increasingly impossible as her mother-in-law demanded attention all the time. Mrs Patel senior was diagnosed with dementia five years ago. She had been the person who ran the household, so her daughter-in-law could help her husband in the family business. The older Mrs Patel had arrived with her husband as a young woman from Uganda and they had set up the supermarket business. Her husband had died ten years previously. As the dementia progressed, she became less and less able to the point that she could not be left on her own because she would try to do household chores leaving the gas on, taps running, and the front door wide-open. She was also incontinent. She was offered a day care place and she went twice a week for a month to see if it suited her. She was picked up in a minibus at 9.30am and brought home at 3.30pm.

Mrs Patel senior was bewildered by the day centre. She had no idea where she was. The furnishings were modern British in style with a big open sitting/dining area and activity rooms off to the side. She had lost her ability to speak and read English so the signage made no sense since it was all words with no pictures. This was especially difficult, in that one of aims of the day at the centre was to give Mrs Patel a bath or shower and to help her get to the toilet more quickly. None of the spaces was furnished in a way that would have helped her. The place did not smell familiar either, since the food was not what she was used to and none of it was cooked on the premises so there were no food smells. She was distressed all day at the centre and returned home upset. This was very difficult for her family to bear. After the month was up, the situation was reviewed. The staff said it was hard to provide a familiar environment to someone who came from a very different culture. They would have liked to make one of the smaller rooms more appropriate with the help of the family. They would have liked to get a local café to deliver familiar food for Mrs Patel. They wanted signage, especially of the toilet, to have recognisable pictures as well as words.

Box 8.10 Key points: Low cost

- "Familiar" environments are often those we remember most vividly from our teenage and young adult years. Providing this is even more of a challenge when the person with dementia was born overseas
- Smell can be a much neglected aspect of environmental design – yet smells quickly trigger memories and can result in us feeling comfortable or alien
- Signs should have words and pictures. This is crucial for many people with dementia who may be no longer able to read and for people who are illiterate or no longer read English

---

Mrs Forsyth was admitted to a care home in a very fragile state. She had been in an acute hospital with multiple issues including severe breathlessness, severe arthritis, poor circulation, leg ulcers and dementia. She had been at home with a substantial care package until a very severe attack of breathlessness had resulted in a hospital admission. After 14 weeks in hospital, she was assessed as being unable to leave to go home. Mrs Forsyth had run a farm with her husband. When her husband died and her son took over the farm, she had moved into town to be near her daughter. She had lived in a small flat in an extra care complex with a courtyard garden in which Mrs Forsyth spent a lot of time and took an active interest in the plants. The care home was chosen because her daughter liked its hotel style and because it was near enough for her to visit easily after work.

Mrs Forsyth was confined to a wheelchair when well enough to get out of bed, but increasingly it was clear that she was approaching the end of her life. These days most people in care homes have advanced progressive conditions and they should increasingly be seen as places for palliative care (Lakhani 2015). The first floor room she was given was small and the furniture was very limited in part because of the need for a hoist. The window looked out on to the street running alongside the home. She was restless and agitated a lot of the time in spite of excellent palliative care. She lay looking at the sky and talking about needing to feed the animals. She called out for the dog she had had in the past. Ideally Mrs Forsyth needed a room with a wide door to a garden or balcony so her bed could be pushed outside. She needed a view of nature from her window. This was particularly important for her, but in fact, it is a general truth that people nearing the end of life crave contact with nature. She needed something like a dog to stroke. Neville Williams House in Birmingham has many different animals (Fellows and Rainsford 2012). Perhaps a life sized fake collie would have comforted Mrs Forsyth.

Box 8.11 Key points: Low cost

- Remember touch is usually the last sense to go
- Consider what would be suitable for each person

Box 8.12 Key points:

- People from rural areas may yearn for contact with nature
- Similarly people who are dying
- Wide doors to a garden or balcony make it possible to get beds outside
- Views of nature from the bed can be very important

Mr Cryor was admitted to an acute ward following a fall which broke his hip. He was operated on very quickly and taken to an acute ward for the care of the elderly. He was very unwell. His delirium was very stressful to him, his family, the staff and other patients. He was restless; shouting for help, trying to get out of bed and walk, unable to eat or sleep. He was in a bedroom bay with three other men with different conditions. They all had dementia to some degree, but Mr Cryor was the most acutely ill having delirium on top of his dementia. Mr Cryor had nothing to look at from his bed. He would have been much helped by a clock (McCusker et al. 2001) so he could have been orientated to time to some extent. An engaging picture or a good view of nature from his room would have helped (Ulrich et al. 2004) him with his recovery. He had no idea where he was – modern hospitals make no sense to a person for whom a hospital ward was a long room with beds down each side.

Box 8.13 Key point: Low cost

- A big understandable, visible clock is very important for anyone with delirium and/ or dementia. Without it they can be even more disorientated

Box 8.14 Key point:

- A view of nature is known to aid recovery. Something to look at can be a distraction from a very frightening situation

As Mr Cryor recovered, he was able to walk with a walker but he was constantly lost. He was quite unable to find the toilet and was constantly going into storerooms or offices. He was agitated by the constant noise of phones, alarms and loud conversations. He gravitated to the nurses' station where he caused great inconvenience by hanging about and getting in the way. He was constantly being encouraged to go back to his bay. He frequently failed to eat since he neither saw nor understood that the bed table was a dining table with food on it.

Box 8.15 Key points: Low cost

- Toilets should be highly visible with the door painted in contrast to the wall and a big sign. Directional signs may be required. Signs should be at 1.2 metres from the floor
- Doors to staff-only rooms should be painted the same colour as the wall with a high up small sign
- Noise and other over-stimulation, should be minimised

Box 8.16 Key points:

- Nurses' stations are not generally a good idea, since they are the only "active" area. A table within sight of each bay so staff can work with their laptop and a quiet office elsewhere are a better idea
- A day room is important so that patients who can move about have somewhere to go. It can also be a recognisable dining room if necessary. Activities can be made available. However they have to be carefully designed or they look like waiting rooms

---

Conclusion

We can cause unnecessary incompetence and disability for people with dementia by failing to attend to the environment. Although we understand this for ourselves if we put ourselves in the shoes of someone with dementia, we nevertheless frequently fail to act on this understanding. Care staff and clinical staff are used to putting up with the environment provided, rather than seeing it as a crucial non-pharmaceutical intervention. We can also cause distressed behaviour by this failure which is then attributed to the dementia – a rather too easy explanation for a lot of our failings.

Getting it right is not easy since we are designing for the impairments of old age as well as the impairments of dementia. There are no disability requirements (like BS 8300) for this combination. Care and clinical staff often have little power to specify the right environment, but they can change it in small but important ways. There can be cost implications, although this can be too ready an excuse. Therapeutic design often takes second place to essential factors such as infection control and ligature prevention, whereas it is equally important and a balance needs to be struck.

Our mantra ought to be that **buildings and outside spaces are an essential part of treatment.** Too often our buildings and outside spaces make people worse not better.

Many thanks to Kenneth Davidson, Jo Hockley, Sarah Penney and Annie Pollock.

64   *Mary Marshall*

References

Fellows, M. and Rainsford, A. (2012) "Animal assisted activities for people with dementia." Chapter in Gilliard, J. and Marshall, M. (eds) (2012) *Transforming the quality of life for people with dementia through contact with the natural world.* London: Jessica Kingsley Publishers.

Fuggle, L. (2013) *Designing interiors for people with dementia.* Stirling: Dementia Services Development Centre.

Houston, A. (2015) *Dementia and sensory challenges. Dementia can be more than memory.* Glasgow: Life Changes Trust. Available from: https://www.lifechangestrust.org.uk/people-affected-by-dementia/dementia-and-sensory-challenges-booklet.

Lakhani, M. (2015) "Palliative care for everyone with advanced progressive incurable illness." *British Medical Journal,* 350: h605.

McCusker, J., Cole, M., Abrahamowicz, M., Han, L., Podaba, J. and Ramman-Haddad, L. (2001) "Environmental risk factors for delirium in hospitalized older people." *Journal of the American Geriatrics Society,* 49: 1327–1334.

Marquardt, G. (2011) "Wayfinding for people with dementia: A review of the role of architectural design." *Health Environments research and Design Journal,* 4(2): 75–90.

Ulrich, R., Quan, X. and Zimring, C. (2004) "The role of the physical environment in the hospital of the 21st century: a one-in-a-lifetime opportunity." Report to the Centre for Health Design.

Wilkes, L., Fleming, A., Wilkes, B.L., Cioffi, J.M. and Le Miere, J. (2005) "Environmental approach to reducing agitation in older persons with dementia in a nursing home." *Australasian Journal on Ageing,* 24(3): 141–145.

Further reading

Department of Health. (2015) "Health building note 08–02. Dementia friendly health and social care environments." www.gov.uk/government/collections/health-building-notes-core-elements.

Pollock, A. and Marshall, M. (2012) *Designing outdoor spaces for people with dementia.* Stirling: Dementia Services Development Centre.

Part II
Supporting people with dementia

9 Dementia and physical health

Understanding the physical impact of dementia

Graham Ellis and Trudi Marshall

Introduction: dementia as a physical disease

In 2016 for the first time in the UK, dementia became the leading cause of death amongst women. In men it came a close second to coronary heart disease. Why should this be the case? It may reflect improvements in the treatment of coronary heart disease and cancer so that the death rates from these conditions have improved. It also reflects the fact that we have an increasingly ageing population. People are living longer which means they are more at risk of developing those diseases associated with old age. Dementia ranks as the most significant among these. Although dementia is often seen as a psychiatric illness affecting cognition, it has a physical illness burden which can be significant, with effects on balance, mobility, continence, eating and levels of physical activity and ultimately dependence. The perception that it is primarily a cognitive problem may result in dementia being under recognised as a medical diagnosis and receiving less attention and care than it should.

We need to become better at understanding, anticipating and planning for the physical effects of dementia. We also need to have a better understanding of the effects of physical disease on dementia.

Some of the effects of dementia in producing physical symptoms can be predicted through an understanding of the pathophysiology of the disease process on the brain. Some of this is a direct impact of the disease process. As damage accrues, critical areas of function affecting walking, balance, vision, continence, swallowing, appetite and posture for instance will occur as a direct result of the disease process.

The secondary effects on a patient's health that can occur as a consequence of the global impact of the disease can include immobility, muscle atrophy and reduced physical fitness.

In addition, it must be remembered that many dementia patients are ageing physically in parallel with their cognitive problems. Physical problems often coincide with cognitive problems. Importantly, the combination of conditions may alter the approach we choose to take in managing a patient. Balancing treatments in a complex case may require developing treatment goals that are more pragmatic, person-centred or focused on quality of life. The potential benefits of hypertension treatments to prevent problems in ten years must be weighed against the burden of taking tablets in a patient with a prognosis of three to five years.

In the early stages of dementia care, attention focuses on the cognitive and emotional impact for patients and their families. This of course is quite right, but it is important to anticipate the physical effects of dementia in order to address changes as they occur, to recognise disease progression and plan accordingly.

Dementia and its effects on physical health

Dementia affects the physical health of patients through several mechanisms. The first is the direct effect of the dementia process on the nervous system. This shows itself in a few areas with physical symptoms causing impairments of function leading to potential disability.

Box 9.1 Case study

Jenny is an 86-year-old lady with Alzheimer's who falls in her living room. She says that she got up to answer the doorbell.

On reviewing her case medically, the team found a number of issues. She has had arthritis for a number of years. She normally walks with a stick and in her rush to answer the door forgot to use the stick. Due to her blood pressure medication Jenny has a degree of postural hypotension. She should wear compressions stockings but often forgets to put them on. She was warned to take her time getting up but was rushing to answer the door. She also has a degree of clutter in her living room with a number of uneven floor surfaces presenting a trip hazard. When the team assessed her balance and gait she has a shuffling gait (not lifting her feet high enough) that is slightly broad based and unsteady.

The team might choose to address her blood pressure by stopping tablets, use a key safe so that her carers can come into the house without startling her, remove clutter from the living room floor or environment to make the visual cues less confusing for her. She can even be supplied with a different walking aid to reduce the risk and tablet supervision (of a rationalised list of medications).

These approaches have been proven to help reduce the falls risk. However Jenny's poor balance may well be a direct affect of the dementia process. Her ability to remember her tablets (even if addressed through planning and home-care) may continue to be a problem and her ability to recall advice to use the walking aid or take care when getting up from a chair may persist. Jenny's risk then of further falls is not eliminated and in fact as her dementia progresses, increases.

Eating and nutrition

Eating, swallowing and nutritional problems are very common in dementia and often become more marked as the disease progresses. For some patients with short term memory loss, cognition can interfere with eating if the individual forgets the task at hand or is easily distracted. This is often a more marked problem in busy or noisy environments such as those seen in the communal dining halls of care homes.

As the condition progresses, other problems such as apraxia (difficulty with complex tasks) and increasing difficulty with fine motor control can make the use of utensils more difficult. Allowing patients to eat finger food can prove a practical way to ensure a consistent nutritional intake.

Patients can also suffer from forms of agnosia (reduced sensory perception) which may result in reduced taste or smell. Additionally patients may struggle with visual agnosia having difficulty distinguishing food on the plate or distinguishing the plate from the table. Reducing visual clutter and the use of high contrast colours are thought to help in these situations.

Chewing and swallowing is a complex physical action. Oral dysphagia is the phenomenon of pocketing food in the mouth. Pharyngeal dysphagia is the problem of triggering a safe swallow. Patients with swallowing difficulties may struggle with aspiration or choking. This can be compounded by oral health problems such as dental decay, poor oral hygiene or swallowing difficulties.

This may result in food or fluids being aspirated in either small or large amounts leading to an increased risk of chest infections. Additionally, superimposed depression (said to be as high as 45% in nursing home residents) may affect appetite or social interaction during dining (Chang 2011).

Sensitive and quiet supportive environments may enhance mealtimes and help to maintain a steady nutritional intake. Eating is a social function and eating in company may help patients to persevere and maintain a dietary intake.

In one study looking at nursing home residents with dementia, those who had eating problems had a 39% six-month mortality rate, making problems with eating in the context of dementia a significant prognostic marker (Mitchell et al. 2009).

Apathy

One common non-cognitive aspect of dementia is that of apathy. Said to affect up to 70% of patients with dementia, the incidence can also vary according to the type of dementia (Cipriani et al. 2014). Apathy in dementia is that phenomenon characterised by an inability to generate or successfully complete a programme of activities, with difficulty initiating actions or thoughts and with a lack of spontaneous activity. Apathy in this context is distinct from depression with its effects on negative thoughts or emotional distress. It is different from dementia related problems of psychomotor slowing and fatigue. Depression is very common in dementia as is fatigue and it is important to distinguish these problems, as depression is potentially amenable to treatment.

Apathy is thought to be a distinct problem caused by damage to the prefrontal and basal ganglia pathways that are associated with motivation and the initiation of executive function.

Apathy is often under recognised in patients with dementia and is associated with functional dependence. There are no safe or truly effective pharmacological treatments for apathy as a consequence of dementia.

Walking and dynamic balance

It is common in patients with dementia to have problems with balance, gait and walking. This reflects the complexity of a task that in some respects we take for granted such as standing, walking or climbing stairs.

Maintaining a standing balance requires proprioception, visual and semi-circular canals input to help you sense whether you are upright, and allow regular adjustments of power in the legs and trunk to maintain position. These sensory inputs need to be managed in a dynamic continuous and co-ordinated way to avoid falling over.

In vascular dementia, specific vascular defects in the motor cortex or internal capsule can affect power. Damage to the cerebellum can affect balance and lesions in the occipital cortex or visual pathways affecting vision. Dementia with Lewy Bodies (DLB) has many symptoms similar to Alzheimer's and Parkinson's disease (Alzheimer Society 2015). People typically experience some Parkinson symptoms including problems with postural stability and gait disorders.

Neurological damage results in a disruption to the complex coordination and planning of movement required to make walking safe. This is seldom sudden and complete, but is often progressive in subtle deterioration that can be seen in a number of ways. Patients with advanced dementia may have difficulty with balance. This may be seen in their walking posture causing them to lean over too far forward or too far back and in more extreme cases can be seen in sitting posture where patients are unable to sit straight upright with a tendency to lean to one side or the other. Patients can lose arm swing, one of the natural balance and corrective movements that allow safe walking. Some patients may shuffle their feet having difficulty lifting and placing them.

Continence

Dementia patients are twice as likely to suffer from urinary incontinence than those without dementia. Again, continence is a complex neurological process requiring sensory input to detect the bladder is full, the suppression of the natural reflex tendency to want to empty the bladder and social awareness to take action and go to the bathroom when required. Awareness of an episode of incontinence can be lost as well as the social ability to recognise the problem.

Faecal incontinence is more usually a sign of advanced disease and is extremely difficult to manage. It can make caring very challenging. Excluding simple things such as constipation with overflow or medication related effects can be important. Medication to help manage incontinence is seldom useful and can be harmful. For instance treatment for urinary incontinence with medication includes anticholinergics to attempt to reduce the bladder stimulus to empty. This can have a detrimental effect, worsening confusion through their centrally mediated anticholinergic action. In general medication should be avoided for the management of urinary incontinence related to dementia. Simple approaches such as regular toileting and measures to maintain patients mobility to get to the toilet and the use of continence products can be effective in preventing or managing incontinence.

Box 9.2 Case study

Audrey has a fall getting up from bed at night. She has difficulty seeing in the poor lighting and is lightheaded when she gets up. She falls in the hall breaking her hip. Her careers find her a few hours later and promptly get her to hospital. She gets surgery for her hip, however Audrey has a prolonged and complicated admission. She develops kidney problems and delirium after the operation. She has difficulty mobilising again. After a long admission it becomes clear that Audrey can no longer safely remain at home. Audrey's family find a care home for her and she is transferred from the hospital to the care home on discharge.

Indirect effects of dementia on physical health

More often physical illness associated with dementia is part of a complex picture and it is hard to draw a direct link. Dependence can occur because of increased problems with self-care, mobilisation or other problems of executive function such as safety awareness and planning (being housebound because of dementia). Associated with dependence is a reduced physical activity resulting in a loss of cardiovascular fitness. It can exacerbate sarcopenia (atrophy of skeletal muscle) and create an increased vulnerability to illness, reduced activity or increased risk of falls.

Falls in older people with dementia are common. Whilst falls may have many causal factors (including postural hypertension, medication side-effects, vision problems) the underlying dementia process can be a significant factor. This is difficult to remedy. Older patients with dementia are at risk of falling with fractures. Colles fractures of the wrist or fractures of the hip are a classical injury for an adult falling from standing height. This is compounded if patients have osteoporosis and therefore, predisposed to fracture.

Medication

Due to comorbidities, patients with dementia have a higher likelihood of being on multiple medications. This may be appropriate for the management of multiple conditions however, as the number of medications increases several consequences ensue. Increasingly complex drug regimes and multiple medications are known to be correlated with poor levels of patient concordance. Secondly the risk of drug side effects is increased as more medications are consumed. Finally drug interactions become more likely as the number of medications increases.

In addition, people with dementia may have an increased susceptibility to side-effects of common medications. Some medications can have centrally acting side-effects. An example is medications that have an anticholinergic side-effect which can exacerbate cognitive decline. Other medications such as analgesics, opiates or sedatives can also have an increased centrally acting impact leading to adverse outcomes (Fox et al. 2011).

Dementia in association with physical disease

More adults surviving into old age means that as the population ages, older adults have a rising number of co-morbidities (see Figure 9.1). Dementia may overlap with other conditions such as chronic obstructive pulmonary disease, diabetes, ischaemic heart disease, hypertension, stroke etc., and this makes dealing with an individual more complex.

A review of primary care patients in the UK found that only 5.3% had dementia as a sole diagnosis. Those over 65 with Dementia had on average 4.6 other chronic conditions (Guthrie et al. 2012). This included Ischaemic Heart Disease (21%), stroke (18%), diabetes (13%), Chronic Obstructive Pulmonary Disease (9%), heart failure (6%) and depression (32%).

The older population is a diverse group. Many older people are fit and active whilst some are vulnerable and require help with self care for example. It is also apparent that some older people can very quickly tip from their position of independence to a position of dependence with only minor triggers. This vulnerability is called frailty: the idea that an individual is vulnerable to catastrophic or sudden loss of function in the context of an acute illness or injury. Co-morbidities seem to be an increasing risk factor for frailty, as is age itself.

Understanding and describing this state of increased vulnerability to a poor outcome is useful in helping target treatments to avoid loss of function, dependence or nursing home admission. Although frailty is largely a physical illness concept it is recognised that dementia and frailty overlap significantly. Dementia patients are more at risk of

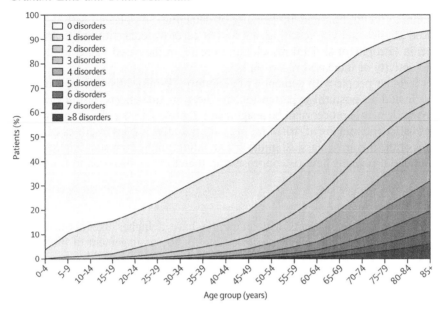

Figure 9.1 The prevalence of comorbidities with age
Source: Barnett et al. (2012).

sudden decline in physical health and loss of function when affected by illness. In that sense dementia is a significant potential component of the frailty syndrome.

Frailty, therefore, more than age or physiological parameters best identifies when an older person is at risk of a disability from an acute illness. Assessment of frailty is essential if an older person is to receive targeted interventions.

Older people are more prone to the complications of disease. The risk is increased across multiple domains such as adverse drug reactions, surgical wound infections, delirium, malnutrition, falls, pressure sores, venous thrombo-embolism, hospital acquired infections, constipation and deconditioning.

Treatment plans for an older adult will often include parallel aims such as the treatment of an acute infection, the rehabilitation of functional decline, the palliation of cancer-related pain and the support for a chronic disease such as diabetes.

The likelihood of multiple overlapping problems necessitates assessment across multiple domains to develop a multifaceted therapeutic plan for recovery and independence. This approach to care involves assessing a patient presenting with an urgent problem across several domains such as physical health, activities of daily living, mental and emotional health and mobility. Different members of the multi-disciplinary team may identify simultaneous problems (such as falls, poor mobility, pneumonia and delirium) and collaboratively coordinate care for the patient that might include medication, rehabilitation and planning of care needs.

This process is referred to as Comprehensive Geriatric Assessment or CGA. CGA is a highly evolved form of ongoing care led by doctors, nurses and allied health professions (physiotherapy, occupational therapy, speech and language therapy, dietetics) who specialise in looking after older adults with frailty and work as a coordinated multidisciplinary team. This may be delivered in a specialist ward or by a mobile team in other areas of medicine or surgical care.

Comprehensive Geriatric Assessment applied to older people with frailty, including those with dementia improves clinical outcome (reduces mortality and the need for long-term care) and reduces the burden of health and social care.

This process needs to be iterative as patients' needs may change, and requires specialist knowledge and clear coordination of care. Ultimately the planning of the individual's care needs to be realistic and patient centred.

Physical illness and its adverse effect on dementia

Individuals who are physically unwell and have dementia are at increased risk of delirium. This risk is significantly higher than in the general population without dementia. Delirium can accentuate the long term cognitive state of the patient.

Delirium (see Chapter 18) is characterised by disturbed consciousness, cognitive function or perception (including hallucinations), and has an acute onset and typically fluctuating course.

It is a serious condition that is associated with poor outcomes including longer hospital stays, more hospital-related complications, such as falls and pressure sores and more likelihood of needing to be admitted to long-term care from hospital.

Dementia and surgical risk

Dementia patients may require surgery either as an emergency or electively. The impact of dementia can change the balance of burdens and benefits from surgery.

Box 9.3 Case study

Susan has been in the nursing home for eight months when the carers contact the family. She is now chair or bed bound has lost interest in food. She requires a carer to help feed her at every meal. Sometimes she seems to cough when eating. She has been losing weight. She struggles to stand up from chair and now requires a hoist. The family discuss Susan's condition with the GP and the nursing home. They agree that they would want to prioritise Susan's quality of life and do not want aggressive or uncomfortable treatment options for her. They wish her to remain in the nursing home as she gets frailer and construct an anticipatory care plan for her. Several weeks later Susan develops a chest infection and passes away quietly in her sleep.

Dementia patients have higher post operative lengths of stay, higher incidence of delirium and immobility post operatively and a greater need for post operative rehabilitation.

Anywhere between 10% and 50% of people having surgery develop delirium and the rates are higher in those with dementia. Functional decline and immobility complicate post operative recovery. Where cooperation with therapists and retention of learning is required, this may be challenging and requires careful care planning.

Ultimately post operative patients are also at higher risk of institutionalisation. For elective surgery, whilst the risk of serious adverse effects can be related to the severity of surgery, even minor challenges such as a general anaesthetic can increase the risk of delirium as they can affect neurotransmitter balance.

Therefore before patients are considered for elective surgery, careful consideration should be given to the reasons for surgery, the impact on quality of life for the patient and the potential risks. In some cases this may mean the considerations of alternative strategies to avoid surgery.

Conclusion

Physical illness treatments and management need framed in the wider context of the dementia. A balance sometimes has to be reached between treatments that prolong life and those that promote comfort and retain dignity where possible. In the medical literature, many carers prioritise comfort over life prolonging treatment. Some treatments such as tube feeding in advanced dementia are now actively discouraged as adding little benefit to the patient and creating potential harm.

Hospitalisation too can be a burden at the end of life. Anticipatory plans developed with carers may encapsulate a patient's wishes and prevent inappropriate treatments in the late stages of dementia.

It is essential that the person and family members take time early in the disease process to plan and anticipate future challenges, identifying what matters most to them and how the person with dementia would like to receive care in the future as their physical health deteriorates.

For instance aiming to manage symptoms and problems without the need for institutional or hospital care may represent a person's wishes. Planning in patients with specific risks such as falls, problems with nutrition, continence or medication allows these problems to be addressed. Lastly and importantly looking ahead for palliative support becomes possible and problems can be anticipated.

One study of nursing home residents with advanced dementia demonstrated that the patients after an episode of pneumonia had approximately a 50% six-month mortality. Recognising these sentinel events appropriately can potentially avoid inappropriate care or burdensome interventions. Antibiotic use is high in patients in residential care with dementia. Much of this may be inappropriate such as the treatment of presumed UTIs in patients with few symptoms or with little confirmatory evidence.

Generally, in patients who have dementia a multidisciplinary approach is best planning to assess the social environmental physical and functional effects of their illness and to coordinate a plan for treatment.

Ultimately recognising that dementia has a significant physical impact (whether directly caused by the dementia process or indirectly by its association with other diseases), is vital when providing care. This must be treated alongside the cognitive, social and emotional elements of this disease.

References

Alzheimer Society. (2015) "Dementia with Lewy bodies: what is it and what causes it?" Available from: http://www.alzheimers.org.uk/site/scripts/documents_info.php?documentID=113.

Barnett, K., Mercer, S.W., Norbury, M., Watt, G., Wyke, S. and Guthrie, B. (2012) "Epidemiology of multimorbidity and implications for health care, research, and medical education: a cross-sectional study." *The Lancet*, 380(9836): 37–43.

Chang, C.C. and Roberts, B.L. (2011) "Strategies for feeding patients with dementia." *American Journal of Nursing*, 111(4): 36–44.

Cipriani, G., Lucetti, C., Danti, S. and Nuti, A. (2014) "Apathy and dementia. Nosology, assessment and management." *The Journal of Nervous and Mental Disease*, 202(10): 718–724.

Fox, C.L., Richardson, K., Maidment, I.D., Savva, G.M., Matthews, F.E., Smithard, D., Coulton, S., Katona, C., Boustani, M.A. and Brayne, C. (2011) "Anticholinergic medication use and cognitive impairment in the older population: the medical research council cognitive function and ageing study." *Journal of the American Geriatric Society*, 59(8): 1477–1483.

Guthrie, B., Payne, K., Alderson, P., McMurdo, M.E.T. and Mercer, S.W. (2012) "Adapting clinical guidelines to take account of multimorbidity." *British Medical Journal*, 345: e6341.

Mitchell, S.L., Teno, J.M., Kiely, D.K., Shaffer, M.L., Jones, R.N., Prigerson, H.G., Volicer, L., Givens, J.L. and Hamel, M.B. (2009) "The clinical course of advanced dementia." *New England Journal of Medicine*, 361: 1529–1538.

Further reading

Comprehensive geriatric assessment

Ellis, G., Gardner, M., Tsiarchristas, A., Langhorne, P., Burke, O., Harwood, R.H., Conroy, S.P., Kircher, T., Somme, D., Saltvedt, I., Wald, H., O'Neill, D., Robinson, D. and Shepperd, S. (2017) "Comprehensive geriatric assessment for older adults admitted to hospital." *Cochrane Database of Systematic Reviews*, 7. doi:10.1002/14651858.CD006211.pub2.

Comorbidities, polypharmacy and anticholinergic medication

Barnett, K., Mercer, S.W., Norbury, M., Watt, G., Wyke, S. and Guthrie, B. (2012) "Epidemiology of multimorbidity and implications for health care, research, and medical education: a cross-sectional study." *The Lancet*, 380(9836): 37–43.

Fox, C.1., Richardson, K., Maidment, I.D., Savva, G.M., Matthews, F.E., Smithard, D., Coulton, S., Katona, C., Boustani, M.A. and Brayne, C. (2011) "Anticholinergic medication use and cognitive impairment in the older population: the medical research council cognitive function and ageing study." *Journal of the American Geriatric Society*, 59(8): 1477–1483.

Guthrie, B., Payne, K., Alderson, P., McMurdo, M.E.T. and Mercer, S.W. (2012) "Adapting clinical guidelines to take account of multimorbidity." *British Medical Journal*, 345: e6341.

Frailty

Clegg, A.L., Young, J., Iliffe, S., Rikkert, M.O. and Rockwood, K. (2013) "Frailty in elderly people." *The Lancet*, 381(9868): 752–762.

Dementia care

Downs, M. and Bowers, B. (Eds) (2014). *Excellence in Dementia Care: Research into Practice* (2nd Edition). Maidenhead: Open University Press.

Scottish Executive. (2000). "Adults with Incapacity (Scotland) Act." Edinburgh: Stationery Office. Available from: http://www.scotland.gov.uk/Topics/Justice/law/awi.

Scottish Executive. (2007). "The Adult Support and Protection (Scotland) Act." Edinburgh: Stationery Office. Available from: http://www.scotland.gov.uk/Topics/Health/Support-Social-Care/Adult-Support-Protection.

Scottish Government and the Mental Welfare Commission for Scotland. (2011) "Standards of Care for Dementia in Scotland." Edinburgh: Scottish Government. Available from: http://www.scotland.gov.uk/Publications/2011/05/31085414/15.

Scottish Intercollegiate Guidelines Network. (2006) "Guideline 86: Management of Patients With Dementia." Edinburgh, SIGN. Available from: http://www.sign.ac.uk/guidelines/fulltext/86/index.html.

10 General hospital care of people with dementia

Amanda Johnson and Christine Steel

Introduction

The hospital environment can be frightening and disorientating for a person with dementia, particularly as the reason for admission is that they are unwell. Evidence shows that people with dementia who are admitted into hospital experience poorer outcomes including deterioration of functional independence, poorer quality of life, increased mortality and length of stay and the increased likelihood of transfer into a care home on discharge Alzheimer Society 2009; Banks et al. 2014; Bridges and Wilkinson,2011; Cowdell 2010; Mental Welfare Commission for Scotland 2010; NHS Confederation 2010).

Within the UK there is a continued drive to improve outcomes for people with dementia and their families and caregivers when hospital admission is unavoidable, and for the staff who provide care in these settings. In Scotland, human rights-based approaches and a focus on person-centred care underpin all our current policies and legislation in order to firmly focus the rights to quality of care, choice, and equality for those whom we care for.

The sections within this chapter will outline and explore the following four core approaches in order for those supporting people with dementia in hospital settings to feel confident and informed to continue to improve outcomes for those that we care for;

- Understand the illness
- Know the person
- Work in partnership
- Respond sensitively

Throughout the chapter there will be examples of good practice, reflective questions and opportunity to apply the learning within your own practice and workplace.

Understand the illness

Traditionally the general hospital system functions on the assumption that people are able to articulate their wishes, respond appropriately whilst acknowledging the needs of others and flow freely through a busy, chaotic system. However, for a person with dementia, particularly when they are faced with physical illness or injury, being admitted and spending time in hospital can be a very difficult experience during their inpatient stay, as well as the adverse impact it may have on long-term outcomes for both individuals and their families/carers.

At a period of significant complexity and challenge within the system, there is an opportunity to think innovatively, consider demand and capacity, and perhaps more importantly have a better prepared workforce in order to create positive learning experiences for all (Baillie et al. 2012) High patient acuity, quick patient turnaround whilst meeting complex care needs of people with dementia can be extremely challenging for staff and often leads or contributes to negative perceptions (Tadd et al. 2011). It is acknowledged that such cultural and organisational barriers in hospital are significant (Houghton et al. 2016) and require a whole system approach to ensure that everyone involved in the process of delivering care within general hospitals are fully skilled, confident and supported to do so. This is reflected in the Clinical Strategy.

Box 10.1 Key point

[T]he need for a new clinical paradigm that will ensure that healthcare delivery is proportionate and relevant to individual patient's needs and uses minimally disruptive interventions (including lifestyle changes) wherever possible.

(Scottish Government 2016)

In response to educational requirements arising from Scotland's National Dementia Strategy (Scottish Government 2010) Promoting Excellence (Scottish Government 2011) provides a framework that details the skills and knowledge that all staff should aspire to achieve in relation to their role, in order to meet the needs of people with dementia, their families and carers. As such there have been significant achievements in implementation of training against the framework however it is important to consider that in the provision of hospital settings as supportive environments, staff may require further support following training to translate the knowledge and skills they have developed into practice. Furthermore Nilsson et al. (2012) suggest that providing ongoing support to staff promotes positive attitudes to minimise the perceived burden of caring for people with dementia in hospital.

A national Dementia Champions training programme in Scotland has now supported over 700 clinicians who work in or around the hospital interface, and working collectively with Dementia Nurse & AHP Consultants within each Board are key to driving forward improvements around the ten Care Actions (Scottish Government 2010, 2013) at a strategic and operational level. Acknowledging and seeking expertise within your own system for example; local dementia champions, Dementia Nurse/AHP Consultants or specialist nurses may be able to provide further support to ensure that staff feel more informed, resilient and confident whilst actively promoting collaborative working. However as Clarke and Mantle (2016) suggest the dementia champions often experience the same pressures and constraints identified by other staff members therefore it is important to ensure that they are also given the time and support to focus on their role as change agents.

Box 10.2 Reflection

See yourself in everyone you meet:

• Consider how would you feel if you were to be admitted to your ward?
• What would a good day look like to you?

- What do you need to maintain resilience and wellbeing?
- What matters to you?

As well as traditional methods of education, the case study below highlights an innovative approach by a dementia champion to support staff within an acute hospital setting.

Box 10.3 Case study

NHS Fife recognised that their task orientated approach to care within a busy and noisy Emergency Department was impacting on levels of stress and distress for people with dementia. In order to support healthcare professionals to understand the experience of stress and distress in this environment, a teaching resource called the "Dementia Box" was developed and implemented by a Dementia Champion. Staff are asked to rebuild an origami box whilst answering lots of complex questions at the same time. This helped staff understand what stress and distress feels like. As a result, there are increased numbers of ED staff and paramedics now completing the NES elearning Dementia Care in the Emergency Department module and it has led to a more person-centred approach to care with fewer members of staff providing direct care to a person with dementia in the department.

Know the person

Admission to hospital for the person with the dementia is generally for reasons other than dementia, and yet there is the risk that the person's dementia and presentation becomes the main focus for healthcare professionals despite it not being the primary reason for admission. The nature of general hospital care means that admission can and does occur at any stage across the disease trajectory and so incorporates a wealth of possible pathways, such as pre-admission clinics, emergency attendance, elective interventions and outpatient appointments therefore it is little wonder that we often lose the individual in our struggle to keep up with the process.

> Whilst physical safety remains a key focus for healthcare, the ability to maintain self-identity and key relationships is of more importance to the person with dementia and their family.
>
> (Gilmour et al. 2003)

"Knowing about a person is a precursor to caring" and can help to positively inform the care provided (Abley 2013). However, gathering a personal history about the person with dementia including their likes and dislikes, is not routinely collected when the person is admitted into hospital (Baillie et al. 2012).

For healthcare professionals working in a general hospital, using the time spent with the person with dementia during physical task orientated care as an opportunity to focus on becoming more "person-centred in their practice" (McCormack 2004) might help staff to see that person-centeredness can be incorporated into their normal daily activities and does not always require more time.

Early conversations to understand the person's lived experience, existing supports and important relationships, what keeps them well and the strengths they possess are fundamental from the onset of admission and throughout their hospital stay. This may be achieved using positive dialogue, use of resources such as Getting to know me and "What matters to me" whiteboards and anticipatory care plans.

The Dementia Care Standards in Scotland and the Royal College of Psychiatrists make recommendations on the use of personal profile tools to gather this information and help inform care which is personalised. The use of personal profile tools also provides an opportunity for risk enablement helping support staff to take strengths based approach.

> I felt [Getting To Know Me] it was greatly to her benefit and as far as I could judge it did not take a significant amount of extra time from ward staff. I feel that my mum was calmer during her recent hospital stay and I also felt that staff sought more information from me and as a result her discharge was well planned.
>
> (Caregiver, NHS Highland)

Despite this increased awareness and focus, there are challenges and significant variation in implementing person-centred care to people with dementia in an acute hospital setting (Nilsson et al. 2013) however if we recognise the importance of understanding who and what matters to the person with dementia, we need to ensure that we use the knowledge to inform personalised plans of care. Meaningful conversations with the person with dementia, their families and carers will be key to success.

Box 10.4 Good practice

The Essential 5 Quality Criteria was developed to improve the quality of personalised planning. The five principles clarify the expected minimum level required to evidence a high quality personalised care plan. Although initially developed to support post-diagnostic support it is completely transferable across all settings. The guidance and bundle can be found at ihub.scot. The following case study (Box 10.5) highlights applicability within a hospital setting.

Box 10.5 Case study

John, 75, has Lewy body dementia and delirium. After several weeks in general hospital, he was admitted to a continuing care setting for further assessment, with frequent episodes of stress and distress. John had a Getting to Know Me document however none of the information around who and what matters to him was clearly outlined in his plan of care. One-to-one nursing observations and antipsychotic meds were prescribed. A personalised care plan focusing on strengths and capabilities was developed with John, his daughter and a staff nurse. They subsequently reviewed the care plan against the Essential 5 bundle.

I felt really listened to and then the information acted upon; I also feel that I have a good rapport with staff now and am able to voice any concerns without a problem.

(Family member)

By reviewing the plan against the Essential 5 bundle...we were able to evidence aspects of good personal planning but also where there were gaps for improvement.

(Staff nurse)

Work in partnership

Open and transparent communication, relationships and interactions at all points in the care pathway are imperative to achieving transformational change; yet within the complexity of acute care settings partnership working is often an assumed or over-looked element of practice. Traditional approaches to care can result in a "them and us" culture; with partnership being viewed either in relation to the wider multi-disciplinary team or as applied to the person with dementia, their family, friends or carers. In this sense, delivery of health related interventions remains as the domain of the professional "expert"; while family members, friends and carers are consulted to provide the personal narrative essential to providing individualised care. However, as previous sections have highlighted, improving outcomes for people with dementia in hospital settings relies upon a synthesis of both knowledge and understanding.

Working in partnership with carers is now a central theme across policy and practice within the UK and fundamental to this is an acknowledgment of the added value that families, friends and carers can bring to the therapeutic relationship. Getting to know the individual with dementia is a prerequisite for personalised care and families, friends and carers can offer not only an insight into the individual's current abilities and preferences but also a link to their past biography. By working together to combine expertise and skills, interventions and rehabilitation approaches can be tailored in such a way as to engage both the person with dementia *and* their family member, friend or carer. Valuing this wider experience and knowledge is one of the most powerful ways in which healthcare staff can improve the sustainability of care provided.

Box 10.6 Reflection

What opportunities are there within your daily practice to work in partnership with families, friends and carers?

Box 10.7 Good practice

John's Campaign was founded in November 2014 in England to fully support carers' rights to continue to care for their loved one during their hospital stay. Many NHS Boards within Scotland have now pledged their support to the campaign which is not just the simple concept of allowing open visiting but that carers are welcome and are considered part of the team around the person. Staff can talk to carers about sharing care and ensuring that the appropriate support is provided during their family members stay in hospital.

Admission to hospital can be an unsettling time for family members, friends and carers as well as for the person with dementia. There is a common fear that the identity of the individual will become lost behind the diagnosis and that functional skills will be eroded and this fear is not without foundation. In such a complex and potentially frightening environment, faced with physical illness or injury and working within strict time and financial pressures, it is easy for staff to get caught up in a pattern of promoting safety by "doing to" rather than "doing with". However, an over-reliance on "safety first approaches" can pose a barrier to the person-centred models of care essential to promoting inclusion and autonomy for people with dementia, their families, friends and carers. The concept of risk enablement provides a useful framework to counteract this pattern by supporting staff to reappraise risk to include not only specific harms or hazards (such as falls) but also those domains of activity and engagement essential to promoting quality of life. Going back to the example of falls – a "falls risk assessment" may generate options to safeguard the person from possible injury. Bed rails or chair alarms are typical examples of falls risk reduction strategies put in place when we base our decision making on deficits. But if focus is shifted to promoting quality of life, then risk of falls becomes one possible harm that can then be balanced against a range of other potential positive and negative outcomes. This might include the physical health benefits of maintaining mobility, the psychological benefit that comes from promoting continence or the social benefit of engaging in interaction with their wider environment. In this way, we can start to consider vulnerability as a by-product of the person's situation and solutions can focus on providing a supportive environment for the person to continue to maintain their autonomy.

Box 10.8 Good practice

#endPJparalysis is a campaign which originated from the work of Brian Dolan, Director of Service Improvement at Canterbury District Health Board in New Zealand and has built up considerable momentum on social media. In essence, the campaign focuses on encouraging people to wear their own clothes, rather than hospital gowns or pyjamas unless they need to. At the heart of the campaign is the issue of deconditioning, such as the fact that for people over the age of 80, ten days bed rest equates to ten years of muscle ageing and that this loss of function may be the difference between independence and dependence. Getting patients into their own clothes is intended to support skill maintenance/maximisation within the routine of care provision by encouraging people to continue with their normal daily routines and activities.

Respond sensitively

Previous sections have shown how understanding the illness, knowing the person and working in partnership can help to make admission to hospital a less frightening and more empowering event for people with dementia, their families, friends and carers. However, providing care for people with dementia can also be an emotional experience for health care staff – especially at times when the person with dementia seems to be communicating stress or distress. Responding sensitively to the needs of the individual requires not only use of proactive strategies to overcome avoidable triggers but also an understanding of how to recognise and respond to stress and distress in order to ensure that the rights of people with dementia are respected.

Person-centred care means treating the people we care for with kindness, compassion, dignity & respect. However it is widely recognised that, in addition to the impact of the illness, people with dementia face significant cultural, social and economic barriers to having their rights respected. Documents such as the "Charter of Rights for People with Dementia and their Carers in Scotland" (Box 10.9) (Alzheimer Scotland 2009) use the "PANEL" approach to strengthen the rights of people with dementia and their carers:

Box 10.9 Learning point

Participate in decisions which affect their human rights.
Accountability of those responsible for the respect, protection and fulfilment of human rights.
Non-discrimination and equality.
Empowerment to know their rights and how to claim them.
Legality in all decisions through an explicit link with human rights legal standards in all processes and outcome measurements.

(Taken from Charter of Rights)

Although these may appear to be a "given", if we stop to consider stress and distress as a potential negative consequence of the hospital environment, it raises questions as to how we can claim to uphold the rights of people with dementia. Proactive strategies to adapt the physical environment are one means of attempting to redress the balance and have been found to be more effective when combined with changes to approaches to delivery of care. Simple adaptations to lighting, layout and signage have the potential to reduce falls and distressed behaviour as well as to improve sleep, communication, independence and nutritional intake (Dementia Services Development Centre 2017).

> While there is still room for more evidence supporting environmental adaptation, the evidence we have has shown us that when we adapt the environment to support cognitive impairment, and when those who work within such an environment practice person centred support, it enables people with dementia to live and function better.
> (Dementia Services Development Centre 2017)

Responding sensitively to the needs of the person requires a compassionate, person-centred approach underpinned by reflective practice and an understanding of stress and distress in dementia. Emerging models of care have shown that distressed behaviours are most often an attempt to communicate an unmet need (Cohen-Mansfield, 2000). So, while the way the person acts while they are distressed may be labelled as "challenging" by other people, it is important to recognise the person with dementia may be expressing an emotional state (NES resource). This is particularly useful when considering how we can adapt our own practice to better meet the needs of people with dementia, their family, friends and carers. Kitwood (1997) identified five areas of psychological need that can provide a useful framework for improving outcomes:

- Comfort – the feeling of trust and closeness that comes from others.
- Attachment –finding familiarity and security, particularly in times of change.
- Inclusion – being involved in the lives of others and feeling part of a group/ community.
- Occupation – being involved in the processes of normal life and meaningful activities.
- Identity – knowing who you are and how you feel about yourself.

Hospitals are complex systems and the pressures on care provision are considerable; yet simple changes can have considerable impacts – especially in terms of the quality of life for the person with dementia. The "Hello my name is" campaign is a movement for compassionate care which builds on the need for *comfort* by providing the reassurance required to build trusting relationships, while the Getting to Know me document mentioned earlier can help strengthen the sense of identity by providing truly individualised care. Responding sensitively does not necessarily rely on time intensive, psychological interventions but can often be achieved by simple changes to acknowledge that patients are not simply people hosted within our system, but rather as healthcare professionals we are guests in our patients' lives.

Box 10.10 Good practice

Pocket Ideas – "a moment in time" is an award-winning project created by the "activity team" within the Occupational Therapy service in NHS Ayrshire & Arran. It is an activity tool filled with ready prepared activities to start a meaningful conversation with older people. There are five sections within the tool that include communication, games, physical activity, music and culture and wellbeing. There are also inspirational quotes and pictures throughout the book. Pocket ideas has been designed with the intention that any member of staff or carer could use it, simply pick a page and start that conversation! Even five minutes with an older person can enhance their quality of life and support a person-centred approach to meaningful conversation. The resource pdf can be accessed at www.nhsaaa.net/active lyengaged and additional information can be requested by emailing PocketIdeas@aapct. scot.nhs.uk. The resource will be available nationally across Scotland in the near future.

I had a lady unwilling to wash and dress. I started going through some questions from the book, she soon engaged with me and agreed to personal care.

(Staff)

Great way to help to get to know patients better and find out their individual interests.

(Staff)

The book was great, especially talking about all the Scottish places and people, brought back good memories for my Dad.

(Carer)

Summary/conclusion

Admission to general hospital for people with dementia is not always primarily related to the condition and therefore can result in increasing complexity of assessment, treatment of care and discharge. In order to ensure that people with dementia receive the right care and support at the right time, it is fundamental that all staff working within these settings understand the illness, know the person and are able to respond sensitively to individual needs whilst working in partnership with families/carers and integrated partners.

Population projections suggest that there will be a significant increase in the number of people with dementia, as well as the number of older people with dementia and therefore we need to ensure that our hospital services have the capacity and commitment to support the best possible outcomes. A continued focus on spread and sustainability of good practice will strengthen services to ensure that we are able to measure and demonstrate change over time and reduce the variation in quality, pace and scale of improvement.

Where hospital admission is unavoidable, everyone has a key role to play to ensure that the care experience is safe, coordinated, dignified and person-centred ensuring seamless transitions across care settings for people living with dementia.

References

Abley, C. (2013) "Practice Question- Person-Centred Care." *Nursing Older People*, 25(10): 14.

Alzheimer Scotland. (2009) "Charter of Rights for People with Dementia and their Carers in Scotland." Available from: http://www.alzscot.org/assets/0000/2678/Charter_of_Rights.pdf.

Alzheimer's Society. (2009) "Counting the cost: Caring for people with dementia on hospital wards." Available from: https://www.alzheimers.org.uk/site/scripts/download_info.php?fileID=787.

Alzheimer's Society. (2010) "My name is not dementia: People with dementia discuss quality of life indicators." Available from: https://www.alzheimers.org.uk/download/downloads/id/876/m y_name_is_not_dementia_people_with_dementia_discuss_quality_of_life_indicators.pdf.

Baillie, L., Merritt, J. and Cox, J. (2012) "Caring for older people with dementia in hospital Part two: strategies." *Nursing Older People*, 24(9): 22–26.

Banks, P., Waugh, A., Henderson, J., Sharp, B., Brown, M., Oliver, J. and Marland, G. (2014) "Enriching the care of patients with dementia in acute settings? The Dementia Champions Programme in Scotland." *Dementia*, 13(6): 717–736.

Bridges, J. and Wilkinson, C. (2011) "Achieving dignity for older people with dementia in hospital." *Nursing Standard*, 25(29): 42–47.

Clarke, C. and Mantle, R. (2016) "Using risk management to promote person-centred dementia care." *Nursing Standard*30(28):41–46. DOI: 10.7748/ns.30.28.41.s47

Cohen-Mansfield, J., Dakheel-Ali, M.D. and Marx, M.S. (2009) "Engagement in persons with dementia: the concept and its measurement." *American Journal of Geriatric Psychiatry*, 17(4).

Cowdell, F. (2010) "The care of older people with dementia in acute hospitals." *International Journal of Older People Nursing*, 5(2): 83–92.

Dementia Services Development Centre. (2017) http://dementia.stir.ac.uk/blogs/dementia-centred/ 2017-02-06/living-well-why-adaptive-environments-matter-people-living.

Department Of Health. (2010) "Nothing ventured, nothing gained: risk guidance for people with dementia." https://www.gov.uk/government/publications/nothing-ventured-nothing-ga ined-risk-guidance-for-people-with-dementia.

Gilmour, H., Gibson, F. and Campbell, J. (2003) "Living alone with dementia: a case study approach to understanding risk." *Dementia*, 2(3), 403–420. Available from: http://journals.sa gepub.com/doi/abs/10.1177/14713012030023008.

Houghton, C., Murphy, K., Brooker, D. and Casey, D. (2016) "Healthcare staffs' experiences and perceptions of caring for people with dementia in the acute setting: qualitative evidence synthesis." *International Journal of Nursing Studies*, 61: 104–116.

Jackson, T.A., Gladman, J.R.F., Harwood, R.H., Maclullich, A.M.J., Sampson, E.L., Sheehan, B. and Davis, D.H.J. (2017) "Challenges and opportunities in understanding dementia and delirium in the acute hospital." *PLoS Med*, 14(3).

Kitwood, T. (1997) "The experience of dementia." *Aging & Mental Health*, 1(1): 13–22.

McCormack, B. (2004) "Person-centredness in gerontological nursing: an overview of the literature." *Journal of Clinical Nursing*, 13(1): 31–38.

Mental Welfare Commission for Scotland. (2010) "Dementia: decisions for dignity." Available from: http://www.mwcscot.org.uk/media/53187/Decisions%20for%20Dignity%202010.pdf .

NHS Education for Scotland And Scottish Social Services Council. (2011) "Promoting excellence: A framework for all health and social services staff working with people with dementia, their families and carers." Edinburgh, Scottish Government. Available from: http://www.gov.scot/Resource/Doc/350174/0117211.pdf.

NHS Confederation. (2010) "Acute awareness: Improving hospital care for people with dementia." Available from: http//www.nhsconfed.org.

Nilsson, A., Lindkvist, M., Rasmussen, B.H. and Edvardsson, D. (2012) "Staff attitudes towards older patients with cognitive impairment: need for improvements in acute care." *Journal of nursing management*, 20(5): 640–647.

Scottish Government. (2010) "Scotland's National Dementia Strategy (2010–2013)." Edinburgh, Scottish Government. Available from: http://www.scotland.gov.uk/Publications/2010/09/10151751/0.

Scottish Government. (2011) "Promoting Excellence: A framework for all health and social services staff working with people with dementia, their families and carers." Available from: https://www2.gov.scot/Publications/2011/05/31085332/0.

Scottish Government. (2013) "Scotland's National Dementia Strategy 2013–2016." Edinburgh. Available from: http://www.gov.scot/Topics/Health/Services/Mental-Health/Dementia/DementiaStrategy1316.

Scottish Government (2016) "A National Clinical Strategy for Scotland." Available from: http://www.gov.scot/Publications/2016/02/8699.

Tadd, W., Hillman, A., Calnan, S., Calnan, M., Bayer, T. and Read, S. (2011) "Right place-wrong person: dignity in the acute care of older people." *Quality in Ageing and Older Adults*, 12(1): 33–43.

World Health Organisation (WHO) and Alzheimer's Disease International (ADI). (2012) "Dementia: a public health priority." Geneva, World Health Organisation. Available from: https://www.alz.co.uk/WHO-dementia-report.

Useful websites

http://www.scie.org.uk/dementia/resources/files/working-in-partnership-with-carers.pdf?res=true.
http://johnscampaign.org.uk/#/.
http://www.last1000days.com/.

11 Palliative and end-of-life care

Jenny Henderson and Barbara Sharp

Introduction

The recognition of dementia as a life shortening illness has been slow to evolve beyond specialists in the field and until relatively recently was often overlooked on death certification as either a cause or contributory factor. Although there is increasing recognition of the role of palliative care in dementia, confusion and diversity of opinion remains over when a palliative care approach should be adopted and the terms used to communicate that care (Kydd and Sharp 2015). A palliative approach can be seen as appropriate from the point of diagnosis because dementia is a syndrome associated with life limiting conditions. However, when a person has recently received a diagnosis of dementia, is it helpful to introduce a term that many will associate directly with the end of life? An important consideration, especially when there is clearly a need to discuss living well, possibly for many years ahead. At the same time, a failure to address the progressive nature of dementia and the need for planning ahead in a timely, person-centred fashion, can exacerbate many of the inevitable practical and emotional difficulties to come. The timing of such conversations is critical and individual in nature.

A contributory factor in such tensions lies in the broader understanding of the language surrounding palliative and end-of-life care. Although sometimes used interchangeably, the terms palliative and end-of-life care are not synonymous. A range of associated words in common use, such as, 'terminal care' and 'supportive care' are used without equally common understanding (Hughes et al. 2010). Palliative care philosophy is synonymous with the best of person-centred care (see Table 11.1) and whatever language is used the importance of living a full life *and* making preparations for the end of life are relevant to everyone.

> **Box 11.1 Key point**
>
> Living a full life *and* making preparations for the end of life are important to everyone.

Specialist palliative care has developed over years of caring primarily for people with cancer. The field offers specific expertise to support people with life limiting conditions, including dementia – although until very recently this area was poorly understood, and access to palliative care services by people with dementia extremely limited (Crowther et al. 2013). Evidence of attempts to widen access to palliative care support for those experiencing long-term conditions is now emerging in strategic policy and practice guidance (Scottish Government 2015).

Table 11.1 Palliative care and person-centred care

Palliative care	Person-centred care
Holistic	Holistic
Nurtures personhood	Nurtures personhood
Focus is on what is meaningful to the person, their wishes and preferences	Focus is on what is meaningful to the person, their wishes and preferences
Responsive to social, psychological and spiritual needs	Responsive to social, psychological and spiritual needs
Supports family and friends	Supports family and friends
Relationships and effective communication are central	Relationships and effective communication are central
Affirms life	Affirms life

Dementia as a life shortening illness

Access to palliative care is a legal obligation under United Nations conventions and international associations have advocated this as a human right (World Health Organisation 2015). Palliative care has been demonstrated to offer a co-ordinated and compassionate approach with specific strengths in supporting difficult conversations, ethical decision-making and complex symptom management. There is an indisputable need for such skills in advanced dementia and at the end of life, although the knowledge and application of skills differ and more research is required (van der Steen et al. 2014).

Dementia differs from other life shortening illnesses, such as cancer, in important ways. The time from diagnosis to death tends to be much longer and the pattern of dying follows a less predictable and more gradual course, punctuated by periods of acute ill health (Sachs et al. 2004). As dementia advances, the range of associated physical, psychological, spiritual and social issues can become more complex, more difficult to recognise and respond to effectively (Alzheimer Scotland 2015). Complexities in advanced dementia include the influence of co-morbid conditions and the challenges brought about by severe changes in modes of communication, physical ability and cognitive capacity. These factors are frequently compounded by a lengthy period of frailty and debilitation which may last as long as three to five years and make the recognition of dying itself more complicated (Neuberger et al. 2013).

Box 11.2 Key point

Dementia shortens lives and progresses over time leading to the need for increasingly complex physical and psychological care.

In the last year of life analysing the progression of the illness and responding appropriately is challenging. Attempts at clarity can be seen in a variety of prognostic indicator guides – for example, the Gold Standards Framework Prognostic Indicator Guidance (Royal College of General Practitioners 2011) and the Supportive and Palliative Care Indicator Tool (SPICT) (University of Edinburgh 2017). These guides advocate a process of:

- Recognising a palliative care need.
- Assessing needs and anticipated support.
- Involving the person, family and multidisciplinary team.
- Planning proactive care.

A need to improve the experiences of people with dementia at the end of their lives, and the support to their families, friends and carers, is recognised across international studies. Failure to provide the best possible care has been associated with several factors, including failure to recognise dementia as a life shortening illness (Potter et al. 2013); challenges in recognising advanced states of the illness and dying (Sampson 2010), and failure to identify the need for palliative care until the last days and weeks of life (Harrison et al. 2012).

The pattern of advanced dementia and its association with periods of acute illness creates the potential for repeated hospital admissions. Hospitalisation may be necessary but needs careful consideration and can expose people with advanced dementia to the risk of invasive, distressing interventions at the end of their lives (Marie Curie 2015). With a focus of curative care, admission to an acute hospital may also hinder delivery of effective palliative care. Recent research indicates people with dementia admitted to acute care at the end of life experience poor symptom assessment in relation to delirium, psychological symptoms and pain (O'Shea et al. 2015).

There is a clear body of evidence that pain experienced by people with dementia is frequently poorly recognised and managed (van der Steen 2010). Currently many pain tools are of limited value in assisting recognition and management of pain in people with dementia (Sampson et al. 2015). The blanket adoption of a single pain tool in settings may be especially unhelpful. A pain history is important, as is assessing pain on movement.

Presentation of pain is individual and may be expressed as distress, especially when communication is compromised. People with dementia are vulnerable to the impact of inaccuracy and inconsistency in pain assessment and poor understanding of the complexities of pharmacological choices in the face of age related changes, multiple-morbidity and cognitive impairment (McLachlan et al. 2011). McLachlan et al. (2011) highlight the importance of closely monitored analgesic dose titration and the need for more research in both pharmacological and non-pharmacological interventions.

Multiple changes can be experienced by people with advanced dementia and these may include: bladder and bowel incontinence; much reduced mobility, being unable to walk; increasing difficulty with eating, difficulties in swallowing; an increasing need for support with all aspects of personal care, increasing levels of disorientation and difficulties with recognition (World Health Organisation 2012). The diverse pattern of potential difficulties and multifactorial nature of their causes demands access to a range of expertise.

Hearing the voice of the person: legal and decision making

The shift in ways decisions are made from the mid 20th century paternalistic approach when 'doctor knew best' to the human rights based framework (Human Rights Act 1998) where thinking is focused on the autonomy of the person can be difficult to achieve for people with dementia. The paternalistic approach was based on the doctor knowing the person. Modern medicine does not always allow for this luxury and relies on the person's residual capacity, the role of proxy decision makers, developing meaningful advance care plans and having open and honest conversations about the life limiting nature of dementia.

A plethora of principles help underpin informed decision making (e.g. Hippocratic Oath, human rights legislation, professional codes of conduct in the UK). However, the impact of dementia clouds decision making, resulting in several high-profile cases where neglect and lack of afforded dignity were evident. Research in Scotland showed proxy decision makers often lacked information and didn't feel supported to use the principles of the legislation under which they were acting (Alzheimer Scotland 2012). A further study identified a variety of emotional and practical factors making proxy decision making difficult for family members (Livingston, et al. 2010).

Advance care planning is important, not only for the person with dementia but for those who may be making decisions on their behalf in the future. Having more information helps to make more informed decisions. Planning avoids leaving unresolved problems for others to grapple with and can provide direction in ensuring ethical informed decision making. Despite these obvious advantages, significant challenges to ensuring advance plans are in place remain:

- Difficult to decide when planning discussions should take place
- Timing of diagnosis – it may be too difficult for the person to contemplate when diagnosis comes early and if late, issues with capacity are likely
- Preferences change as dementia progresses
- It can be hard for people to comprehend future needs
- Families may be expected to address whilst emotionally overwhelmed
- Often addressed as a single activity rather than a process
- No consistent approach to format, location and accessibility
- Professionals may feel ill-equipped to conduct these emotive conversations.

Box 11.3 Key point

Hearing the voice of the person is perhaps one of the biggest challenges. Failings arise when the person lacks or is perceived to lack any decision-making powers and is deemed to lack *all* capacity where in reality we must always presume that there is residual capacity.

Where people with dementia die and how we can promote a good end to life

The recent landscape of care provision for older people with dementia has been changing significantly in association with the ageing demographic. For example, up to a quarter of hospital beds in the UK are occupied by people with dementia over 65 years of age (Alzheimer's Society 2009). In care homes residents are older and much frailer than previously, often experiencing multiple morbidities. All this means that the care of people with advanced dementia and those who are dying is increasingly "everyone's business."

When planning for the future, people with dementia state they would like to die either at home or in their usual place of residence (Marie Curie 2015). Research indicates that for the majority of people with dementia across Europe, dying at home remains relatively rare compared to other settings (Houttekier et al. 2010).

While many people indicate that, in ideal circumstances, home is their preferred place to be cared for when dying, "home" is also described as more than merely a physical place – it is a place of connection, associated with the presence of loved ones (Gott et al. 2004). The continuity of care and connections is vital to the quality of all care and especially so at the end of a person's life. As such, an emphasis on supporting family members and other carers who are already an integral part of the lives of people dying with dementia, and who know them best, is essential.

Box 11.4 Reflective thought

If death can be good...then it would be at home with your family and a staff group that love and cherish you, to hold your hand and to comfort you and your family.

(Manager of a specialist dementia supported housing unit)

Care homes, "care at home" services and housing providers have an increasingly important role to play in caring for people at the end of their lives. When positive relationships are nurtured and staff, friends and family achieve true partnership in support then the best of care can flourish.

Box 11.5 Case study

We were particularly grateful that the staff were able to care for our mother throughout the difficult days of her final illness, allowing her to die in her home surrounded by the caring staff and her family.

(Family members of a person with dementia who died in a specialist dementia supported housing unit that she called "home")

Box 11.6 Key point

Grief is a complex and continually changing process and impacts on the experience of dementia. People respond to and cope with grief in different ways.

Recognising the impact of loss and grief for people with dementia and their families and friends

Dementia is an illness in which loss plays an inextricable part. The impact of grief in dementia has been described by Doka as "a constant but hidden companion" (Doka 2005, 290). The anticipation and impact of losses for both the person with dementia and their family during the illness, and for the family after death are profound.

For each person the experience of loss is unique but there are common themes. A family member may anticipate the death or loss of the person before it occurs. This anticipatory grief also has resonance for people with dementia. A further perspective on grief experienced prior to the physical death of a person has been described as ambiguous loss, reflecting the unclear loss associated with how the person with dementia has changed (Doka 2002).

Some people can accept the changes that have occurred in the person and deal with the situation as it is. Others know the loss has occurred but do not accept it and avoid dealing with the reality – this may impact on family relationships (Dupuis 2002).

> **Box 11.7 Key point**
>
> How families cope with their own losses will influence how they support their family member with dementia and cope with their bereavement.

How the death of someone with dementia is perceived by society can also influence how well the bereaved person copes with their loss. A person's grief that is not being acknowledged by others has been described as disenfranchised grief (Doka 2002). This is experienced when, for example, words of "comfort" such as, "It's a blessing in disguise," are offered, or where the death is not acknowledged at all. Such responses can leave the family member to grieve on their own, feeling the person's life was not valued by others. There is growing recognition of the importance of spirituality and its relationship to wellbeing. However, confusion remains about the concept and the sense of well-being it may provide when attended to. Spirituality forms a core theme in models of care, yet anecdotally plans are rarely well documented or implemented. There is little research as to why this is but a recent study of Norwegian nurses suggests an association between nurses' sense of comfort in completing spiritual assessments, their education on the subject and the level of importance they attribute to it (Cone and Giske 2017). Spiritual *life* can be said to be the essential core which brings meaning, hope and purpose to life (MacKinlay and Trevitt 2006). Spiritual *care* is about tapping into these concepts however the individual may express them.

In advanced dementia physical care may become increasingly unwelcomed by the person with dementia for a variety reasons. These include the presence of pain, fatigue, sensory changes, misinterpretation, limited communication, stress and distress or possibly past abusive experiences. Difficulties may be compounded by care which is task orientated, risk averse and focused on deficits. Creative solutions to maintaining personal care with sensitivity and compassion can be enhanced by person-centred and relationship-centred approaches that focus on strengths, abilities and what really matters to the person with advanced dementia. The following vignette provides an example of such approaches:

> **Box 11.8 Case study**
>
> Jane is an 80-year-old old lady with advanced dementia recently transferred from acute care to a care home. The acute care team report major difficulties in providing Jane with the level of support she requires with her personal care. One key area of difficulty identified is helping Jane to wash her hair and on arrival her hair looks dirty and unkempt. The hospital described how Jane had become very distressed when

they attempted to wash her hair with a shower attachment whilst she was bathing. She was described as "screaming and flaying her arms about, hitting out at staff".

Getting to know the person

The care home team sought background information from Jane's daughter, Elsie, who was able to tell them that Jane never used a shower at home, only ever had a bath. Elsie explained that Jane would wash her hair by leaning over a large sink and this was always carried out separately from her bathing routine. Elsie noted that Jane had always disliked water running down her face and this had become more evident. For years Jane had cleansed her face rather than using soap and water – and she had wonderful skin as a result!

Understanding the difficulties and focusing on what matters

Using a "hand under hand" approach, staff were able to support Jane to cleanse her face without water and applying a moisturising cream (identified by Elsie as a favourite of her mum's). Jane reacted with pleasure to the scent and feel of the cream as she was re-introduced to a familiar routine. Gradually, the care team were able to introduce shampooing Jane's hair into this routine, using products that required no water. Jane seemed relaxed as the product was gently massaged onto her head and again a 'hand under hand' approach was used to support her brushing her own hair. Staff worked with Elsie to help her understand these techniques and she soon adopted some of the routines into her visits to her mum, making their time together much more positive and meaningful.

A key to success in the example provided above is bringing the knowledge, ideas and skills of staff and family together with their shared understanding of the experience and preferences of the person with dementia. The approach illustrated also acknowledges the importance of the senses in later dementia – to care giving, communication and making connection with the person with dementia. A sensory care approach developed within care homes entitled "Namaste Care" has been demonstrated effective in reducing agitation, improving communication and enhancing care giving relationships (Stacpoole, et al., 2015). This approach has recently been adapted and applied in different settings, including a day support facility, where a small-scale study reported that family members and staff perceived a positive contribution to the quality of life of some participants with advanced dementia (Tolson et al. 2015).

Box 11.9 Case study

The first time I worked with this lady I read in the notes that she really relaxed if she had her hair brushed so ... I just sat their brushing her hair and I realised that was a little wee magic moment because she just fell asleep.

(Care worker, day support service)

Shared learning for change

An exciting recent development has been work by a European collaborative to provide a positive practice approach to the support of people with advanced dementia not yet requiring end-of-life care but with increasing needs. The Palliare (to cloak in support) project draws on a biopsychosocial and spiritual model of dementia care that places the person and caring relationships at the centre of healthcare practice. The approach is informed by a literature review on advanced dementia care and family caring, a review of current dementia policies and in-depth case studies on the experience of advanced dementia care and family caring. Four inter-professional accredited learning modules have been developed which focus on equipping the qualified workforce to improve advanced dementia care. Outputs from this project include a "Dementia Palliare Best Practice Statement" (Homerova et. al. 2016) and the establishment of a community of practice (University of West of Scotland 2015).

Box 11.10 Case study

The team looked after our mum with real genuine affection, patience and humour whilst always maintaining true professionalism and being cogniscent of her dignity at all times.

(Family of a person with dementia who died in a specialist dementia supported housing unit)

Acknowledgement

We are grateful to the staff and families of residents in Alzheimer Scotland's Croftspar Place, for permission to use their quotes. Croftspar Place is a small supported housing unit for people with dementia in Glasgow, Scotland.

References

Alzheimer Scotland. (2012) "Dementia: making decisions. A practical guide for family members, partners and friends with powers of attorney, guardianship or deputyship." Available from: http://www.alzscot.org/assets/0000/5331/Dementia-Making-Decisions.pdf.

Alzheimer Scotland. (2015) "Advanced Dementia Practice Model: understanding and transforming advanced dementia and end of life care." Available from: http://www.alzscot.org/news_and_comm unity/news/3462_advanced_dementia_practice_model.

Alzheimer's Society UK. (2009) "Counting the cost: caring for people with dementia on hospital wards, London." Available from: https://www.alzheimers.org.uk/download/downloads/id/787/counting_the_cost.pdf.

Cone, P.H. and Giske, T. (2017) "Nurses' Comfort Level with Spiritual Assessment: A Study among Nurses Working in Diverse Healthcare Settings." *Journal of Clinical Nursing*, 26(19–20): 3125–3136. Available from: https://doi.org/10.1111/jocn.13660.

Crowther, J., Wilson, K. C., Horton, S. and Lloyd-Williams, M. (2013) "Compassion in health-care – lessons from a qualitative study of the end of life care of people with dementia." *Journal of the Royal Society of Medicine*, 106(12): 492–497.

Doka, K.J. (2002) *Disenfranchised grief: New directions, challenges and strategies for practice.* Champaign Illinois: Research Press.

Doka, K.J. (2005) *Living with Grief: Alzheimer's Disease.* Washington DC:Hospice Foundation of America: 290.

Dupuis, S.L. (2002) "Understanding ambiguous loss in the context of dementia care: Adult children's perspectives." *Journal of Gerontological Social Work*, 37(2): 93–115.

Gott, M., Seymour, J., Bellamy, G., Clark, D. and Ahmedzai, S. (2004) "Older people's views about home as a place of care at the end of life." *Palliative Medicine*, 18(5): 460–467.

Harrison, N., Cavers, D., Campbell, C. and Murray, S.A. (2012) "Are UK primary care teams formally identifying patients for palliative care before they die?" *British Journal of General Practice*, 62(598): e344–e352.

Homerova, I., Waugh, A., MacRae, R., Sandvide, A., Hanson, E., Jackson, G., Watchman, K. and Tolson, D. (2016) "Dementia Palliare Best Practice Statement." University of the West of Scotland.

Houttekier, D., Cohen, J., Bilsen, J., Addington-Hall, J., Onwuteaka-Philipsen, B.D. and Deliens, L. (2010) "Place of death of older persons with dementia. A study in five European countries." *Journal of the American Geriatric Society*, 58(4): 751–756.

Hughes, J.C., Lloyd-Williams, M. and Sachs, G.A. (Eds.) (2010) *Supportive Care for the Person with Dementia.* New York: Oxford University Press.

Human Rights Act UK. (1998) Available from: http://www.legislation.gov.uk/ukpga/1998/42/contents.

Kydd, A. and Sharp, B. (2016) "Palliative care and dementia – A time and place?" *Maturitas*, 84: 5–10.

McLachlan, A.J., Bath, S., Naganathan, V., Hilmer, S.N., Le Couteur, D.G., Gibson, S.J. and Blyth, F.M. (2011) "Clinical pharmacology of analgesic medicines in older people: impact of frailty and cognitive impairment." *British Journal of Clinical Pharmacology*, 71(3): 351–364.

Marie Curie. (2015) "Living and dying with dementia in Scotland: Barriers to care." Available from: https://www.mariecurie.org.uk/globalassets/media/documents/policy/policy-publications/february-2015/living-and-dying-with-dementia-in-scotland-report-2015.pdf Accessed 06/04/2016.

Livingston, G., Leavey, G., Manela, M., Livingston, D., Rait, G., Sampson, E., Bavishi, S., Shahriyarmolki, K. and Cooper, C. (2010) "Making decisions for people with dementia who lack capacity: qualitative study of family carers in UK." *British Medical Journal*, 341: c4184.

MacKinlay, E. and Trevitt, C. (2006) "Facilitating spiritual reminiscence for older people with dementia: A learning package." Center for Ageing and Pastoral Studies, St Mark's Theological Centre.

Neuberger, J., Guthrie, C. and Aaronovitch, D. (2013) "More care, less pathway: a review of the Liverpool Care Pathway." Department of Health, UK.

O'Shea, E., Timmons, S., Kennelly, S., de Siún, A., Gallagher, P. and O'Neill, D. (2015) "Symptom assessment for a palliative care approach in people with dementia admitted to acute hospitals results from a national audit." *Journal of Geriatric Psychiatry and Neurology*, 28(4): 255–259. Available from: https://doi.org/10.1177/0891988715588835.

Potter, J.M., Fernando, R. and Humpel, N. (2013) "Development and evaluation of the REACH (recognise end of life and care holistically) out in dementia toolkit." *Australasian journal on ageing*, 32(4): 241–246.

Royal College of General Practitioners. (2011) "Gold Standards Framework Prognostic Indicator Guidance." Available from: http://www.goldstandardsframework.org.uk/cd-content/uploads/files/General%20Files/Prognostic%20Indicator%20Guidance%20October%202011.pdf

Sachs, G.A., Shega, J.W. and Cox-Hayley, D. (2004) "Barriers to excellent end-of-life care for patients with dementia." *Journal of General Internal Medicine*, 19(10): 1057–1063.

Sampson, E. L. (2010) "Palliative care for people with dementia." *British Medical Bulletin*, 96(1): 159–174.

Sampson, E.L., White, N., Lord, K., Leurent, B., Vickerstaff, V., Scott, S. and Jones, L. (2015) "Pain, agitation, and behavioural problems in people with dementia admitted to general hospital wards: a longitudinal cohort study." *Pain*, 156(4): 675–683.

Scottish Government. (2015) "Strategic Framework for Action on Palliative and End of Life Care." Available from: http://www.gov.scot/Topics/Health/Quality-Improvement-Performance/peolc/SFA.

Stacpoole, M., Hockley, J., Thompsell, A., Simard, J. and Volicer, L. (2015) "The Namaste Care programme can reduce behavioural symptoms in care home residents with advanced dementia." *International Journal of Geriatric Psychiatry*, 30(7): 702–709.

Tolson, D., Watchman, K., Richards, N., Brown, M., Jackson, G., Dalrymple, A. and Henderson, J. (2015) "Enhanced Sensory Day Care Developing a new model of day care for people in the advanced stage of dementia: a pilot study." Technical Report, University of the West of Scotland. doi:10.13140/RG.2.1.1474.2568.

University of Edinburgh. (2017) "Supportive and Palliative Care Indicators Tool." Available from: http://www.spict.org.uk/the-spict/.

University of West of Scotland. (2015) "Dementia Palliare, Community of Practice." Available from: http://dementia.uws.ac.uk/

World Health Organisation. (2012) "Dementia: a public health priority." Available from: http://www.who.int/mental_health/publications/dementia_report_2012/en/.

World Health Organisation. (2015) "Fact sheet on palliative care." Fact sheet N°402, July. Available from: https://www.who.int/news-room/fact-sheets/detail/palliative-care .

van der Steen, J.T. (2010) "Dying with dementia: what we know after more than a decade of research. "*Journal of Alzheimer's disease*, 22(1): 37.

van der Steen, J.T., Radbruch, L., Hertogh, C.M., de Boer, M.E., Hughes, J.C., Larkin, P., Francke, A.L., Jünger, S., Gove, D., Firth, P. and Koopmans, R.T. (2014) "White paper defining optimal palliative care in older people with dementia: a Delphi study and recommendations from the European Association for Palliative Care." *Palliative Medicine*, 28(3): 197–209.

Further reading

Anandrajah, G. and Hight, E. (2001) "Spirituality and medical practice: using the HOPE questions as a practical tool for spiritual assessment in office practice." *American Family Physician*, 63: 81–88.

City of Hope Pain and Palliative Care Resource Centre. Available from: http://www.caringcommunity.org/helpful-resources/models-research/city-of-hope-pain-and-palliative-care-resource-center/.

Hughes, J.C., Jolley, D., Jordan, A. and Sampson, E.L. (2007) "Palliative care in dementia: issues and evidence." *Advances in Psychiatric Treatment*, 13(4): 251–260.

Irish Hospice Foundation. (2016) "Loss and Grief in Dementia Guidance, Document 3." Available from: http://hospicefoundation.ie/wp-content/uploads/2016/07/Final-Guidance-Document-3-Loss-Grief.pdf.

12 Legal and ethical issues

Donald Lyons

Introduction

One of the most difficult questions I have been asked is: "Can this person with dementia make his/her own decisions?" The usual answer is, "It depends".

Answering this question requires some understanding of broad aspects of human rights and disability law. Regardless of the law in individual countries and states, there are some overarching principles. You may wish to refer to the European Convention on Human Rights (ECHR) (Council of Europe 1950) and the United Nations Convention on the Rights of Persons with Disabilities (CRPD) (United Nations 2006) for detailed information.

ECHR has several important articles that confer legally enforceable rights where European states have incorporated the convention into domestic laws, e.g. the United Kingdom Human Rights Act (United Kingdom Parliament 1998). Important articles include the rights to life, freedom from torture, liberty and private and family life. Some of these rights can be interfered with but with strict conditions attached. For example, an individual with dementia may lose the right to liberty in order to provide safe care. But he/she must have the right of appeal and there must be periodic external review. Likewise, there can be interference with the right to private and family life, but only if necessary, proportionate and legal.

The CRPD also asserts a number of rights. Many of these are similar to ECHR, but they specifically include the right to independent living and the right to the highest attainable standard of health. Countries, including the UK, that have signed up to the convention must ensure that their legislation complies with the convention. At the time of writing, there is considerable debate about article 12 which asserts the right to equal recognition before the law, including equal "legal capacity". The United Nations Committee that oversees the operation of the convention has called on all states to repeal all laws on involuntary treatment and guardianship, based on its interpretation of article 12 (United Nations Committee on the Rights of Persons with Disabilities 2014). Many other ethical experts have questioned this interpretation (Freeman et al. 2015). It is beyond the scope of this chapter to give a detailed analysis of what this argument means for people with dementia. But it is likely that certain overarching principles will emerge and should, in any case, be uppermost in our ethical framework when approaching the care of individuals with dementia. These are:

- the right to exercise one's own capacity and choice;
- the right to support in decision-making, with substitute decision-makers only where necessary;
- the right not to be subject to restraint and deprivation of liberty unless fully justified and with appropriate safeguards.

Capacity and choice

Firstly, there is a presumption in favour of capacity. Be careful about this. It does not mean that the person has capacity unless you have a piece of paper in your hand that says otherwise. It means that you start from the position that the person with dementia has the capacity to make his/her own decisions. But this presumption can be challenged if you have evidence that the person's ability may be impaired. If so, you must assess, or arrange someone else to assess, the person's capacity. In law, this is called a "rebuttable presumption in favour of capacity".

Secondly, you must be aware that capacity is decision-specific and time-specific. The person may be capable of making some decisions, but not others. He/she may also be capable of making these decisions some of the time, but not all of the time.

Thirdly, where the person does not have capacity, you should still act in a way that is in keeping with the person's wishes. You should only go against the person's wishes if you can demonstrate that this will result in harm to the person or to others. While the principle of taking account of the person's wishes is written into many legislative frameworks, it is usually not expressed as clearly as in article 12 of the CRPD. The laws in England and Wales, Scotland and Northern Ireland follow these principles to varying extents. The Essex Autonomy Project (University of Essex 2016) has useful analysis and guidance on this.

While legal definitions of capacity or incapacity differ among jurisdictions, some fundamentals remain. In order to have capacity in relation to decisions about finance, property, welfare or care and treatment, the person must be able to:

- understand the information relevant to the decision
- retain the information for at least long enough to make a decision
- weigh, balance and question the information
- arrive at a decision and communicate it
- understand the consequences of a decision
- act independently on the decision, where necessary.

So capacity does not depend on whether or not you agree with the outcome. It depends on the process that the person with dementia uses to arrive at a decision. If you think the person lacks capacity, remember that it must be the dementia that interferes with the process of arriving at the decision. It may be helpful to think about what decision the person may have made before he/she might have made before the onset of dementia.

Box 12.1 Case study

Michael has a diagnosis of dementia of Alzheimer type. He cannot remember information given to him after five minutes. He is examined by a dentist who tells him he might need fillings to prevent future decay. He refuses treatment, but the dentist thinks it is still warranted. In the past, Michael rarely went to his dentist and expressed a dislike of having anything done to his teeth unless he was in pain. While it is likely that Michael lacks capacity in relation to the proposed treatment, the dentist must take account of his present and past wishes. If Michael is in pain, or developing a condition such as an abscess that will cause serious future problems, the dentist should intervene, making sure that any intervention is lawful. Otherwise, Michael's refusal of treatment should be respected in line with evidence of past wishes.

Even if the person with dementia cannot remember decisions, you should look at consistency of decision-making and the person's past wishes. The person may have difficulty recalling decisions, but if he/she makes the same decision consistently and/or agrees with the decision when presented with a record of it, then it is likely that, on the basis of memory, he/she has capacity.

Box 12.2 Case study

Saskia is in her eighties and has been diagnosed as having vascular dementia. She has always had a close relationship with her son. She wants him to look after her finances and welfare if she loses the capacity to decide for herself. She is invited to grant power of attorney in favour of her son. After ten minutes, she has forgotten the questions she was asked about this. But when asked again, she is adamant that she wants her son to act for her if she loses capacity. She has some difficulty retaining information, but this does not necessarily impair her ability to decide who she wants to act for her in future.

If her son was previously found to have stolen from her bank account but she does not remember this, this may cast doubt on her ability to decide. But if she does remember this and still wants him to act as her attorney, it is less clear cut. Remember, we can all make unwise decisions. In order to demonstrate incapacity, you have to show that her dementia interferes with her capacity in relation to this decision.

Supported and substitute decisions

International law and conventions require that we do all we can to support the person with dementia to make his/her own decisions. To achieve this, we should:

- Provide the individual with information in a way that best meets their needs. Verbal, written and pictorial information all have their roles depending on the individual. Involvement of experts in speech and language therapy may be valuable in achieving this.
- Give the individual time and support to digest information in order to arrive at a decision. People with dementia are likely to function better in familiar surroundings and may be better at certain times of day, e.g. the morning for individuals with vascular dementia.
- Assist the individual to make his/her own decisions without undue influence. With the best of intentions, relatives and health or social care practitioners may run the risk of imposing their own decisions. There is guidance available on how to do this (Mental Welfare Commission for Scotland 2016).

Despite best efforts, there will be situations where individuals with dementia lack capacity to make some decisions. While the issue of substitute decision-making is controversial, most authorities consider that it is necessary. Safeguards are important. Legal mechanisms differ among jurisdictions but there are common themes:

- Ideally, the individual with dementia should appoint someone to make decisions in the event of future incapacity. This would be in the form of a power of attorney specifying which powers the attorney would have in relation to finances, personal welfare and medical treatment.
- If the individual has not done this, there are common law and statutory precedents for intervening. We all have duties to act out of necessity where intervention is necessary to prevent an individual with dementia coming to harm. *For example, an individual with dementia becomes more impaired as a result of a chest infection. He leaves his house in the middle of the night trying to find his wife who died some years ago. In the absence of specific powers, we have the immediate duty to act to keep him safe by returning him to his house or some other safe place, and to make sure his property and belongings are safe.*
- Substitute decisions on an ongoing basis require a basis in law. Judgements in the UK and European Courts make this clear. This may involve a guardian or other person appointed by a court. Some interventions may not need this level of scrutiny, e.g. medical interventions that are necessary and unopposed and simple measures to use money to pay bills etc.
- But the complicating factor in all of this is the issue of deprivation of liberty. This is dealt with more fully below.

Deprivation of liberty and restraint

The decision to restrain an individual with dementia, or otherwise deprive that person of liberty, is one of the most difficult issues for health and social care practitioners. Yet it is one that requires judgement on a daily basis in many settings.

Box 12.3 Case studies

Mohammed is a man with dementia who has lived alone since his wife died two years ago. He sometimes forgets his wife is dead and goes out looking for her at night and gets lost. He is determined to keep on living independently. What can care practitioners do to help him to stay safe?

Marie has advanced dementia and is in a care home. She walks around the care home constantly, trying locks and exits. She lacks the ability to express where she wants to go, but everyone recognises that she is unsafe to be allowed to leave unescorted. How should they respond?

James has advanced dementia and lacks the understanding of the consequences of his actions. He resides in a care home. He thinks it is his own home and does not understand why other people are there. He shouts and swears at them and attacks them with his walking stick as they pass by. How should staff keep others safe while respecting James as an individual?

All of these cases involve getting a balance between the freedom of the individual with dementia and the risk of harm to that person or others. None has an easy solution. But there are ethical frameworks that can help you, and that are often written into legislation in the form of a set of principles. For example, incapacity legislation in Scotland (Scottish Parliament 1999) has a set of principles that must be applied to any intervention when a person with dementia lacks capacity. Some of these are common to other legislatures and some are expressed differently.

Firstly, any intervention must benefit (or be likely to benefit) the individual. Some jurisdictions use the term "best interests" which is acceptable if you avoid being paternalistic – "we are doing this because we judge it to be in your best interests" does not sound as good as "we are doing this because we think it will benefit you."

Secondly, any intervention to achieve this benefit must the least restrictive of the individual's freedom.

Thirdly, and arguably of particular importance given the CRPD debate, we must take the wishes of the individual into account. These could be present wishes if the person is able to express them. Independent advocacy has an important role here. They could be past wishes, e.g. if recorded in some form of advance directive or values statement, relayed by others who know the individual well, or inferred by knowledge of the individual's lifestyle and previous decisions.

Fourthly, we should consult others if reasonable and practicable to do so. It may be legally necessary to consult an attorney or guardian with proxy powers over significant decisions. But for difficult decisions such as the three above scenarios, getting as many views as possible will help to inform the best way forward.

Finally, it is important to help the individual use existing skills and develop new skills. In the case of the individual with dementia, there is a risk that significant interventions to deprive the person of liberty will result in loss of independent living skills. We should do all we can to guard against this.

The whole issue of authority for deprivation of liberty and restraint is complex. Judgements in national and international courts are inconsistent. Stavert has provided a useful review in relation to the law in Scotland (Mental Welfare Commission 2014) and the Essex Autonomy Project has provided a critique of legislation for England and Wales (University of Essex 2014). Northern Ireland has, at the time of writing, passed bold and progressive legislation that is yet to be tested (Northern Ireland Assembly 2016). Every case is different, so independent advice from a legal and/or ethical perspective is likely to help. In Scotland, the Mental Welfare Commission provides free advice on clinical dilemmas, including options for authorising interventions.

Let us apply these principles to one of the above case scenarios, that of Mohammed. What options exist in relation to his nighttime excursions to try to find his deceased wife? And how do the principles apply, especially in the light of the requirements of ECHR and CRPD as outlined at the beginning of this chapter?

1   Do nothing and hope he does not come to too much harm?
2   Use signs and cues to stop him going out?
3   Sedate him at night so that he sleeps longer and is less likely to go out?
4   Lock his door at night so that he cannot leave?
5   Use technology such as an alarm to alert someone when he leaves the house or provide him with a tag that can track his movements?
6   Have someone stay with him every night?
7   Remove him from his house into a care facility?

Benefit: options 2 through to 7 provide benefit in that they might prevent him coming to harm. But options 3 and 4 carry significant risk of harm. He is alone at home, so falls or accidents caused by sedation could be serious. Locking him in may cause distress and could be dangerous if there is a fire. Option 7 removes his independence. While probably the safest option, is it a proportionate response (right to private life under ECHR)? Options 2 and 5 may be insufficient to ensure his safety. Option 6 may be ideal as long as the presence of someone in his house at night does not distress him. It may unfortunately not be practicable.

Least restriction of freedom: some restriction may be necessary to be of benefit. Option 2 is least restrictive. Technology may be less restrictive that medication or physical barriers, although the restrictions imposed by someone being called out to return him home may cause him distress. Options 3, 4, 6 and 7 are most restrictive.

Views of the individual: Mohammed is less confused during the day so may be able to express a view on how he would prefer to be kept safe at night. It would be best practice to respect his views and act on them unless doing so would be likely to risk harm to him or to others, as per CRPD. For example, Mohammed may ask for his door to be locked at night so that he cannot leave, but this would put him at serious risk if there was a fire.

Consult relevant others: in this case, Mohammed's family live some distance away but are very concerned. He also has concerned and supportive neighbours. We should take account of their views. For example, family members may want Mohammed to go into a care home but this is very much against Mohammed's views.

Existing/new skills: in the case of individuals with dementia, preserving existing skills is the important issue. Option 2, if it works, is most in line with this principle as it helps him to remember not to go out at night.

Ultimately, decisions like this are not easy. Principles and convention articles provide a framework for deciding on interventions. They do not make difficult decisions for us. Try using this framework for the "Marie" and "James" scenarios.

Conclusion

One of the most difficult aspects of care for someone with dementia is deciding whether, when and how to intervene when the individual may have lost capacity. International conventions and domestic laws are complex. But an approach that uses principles based on human rights will help to get the right balance between respecting the individual's wishes and protection from harm.

References

Council of Europe. (1950) European Convention on Human Rights. Available from: http://www.echr.coe.int/Documents/Convention_ENG.pdf.

Freeman, M.C., Kolappa, K., Caldas de Almeida, J.M., Kleinman, A., Makhashvili, N., Phakathi, S., Saraceno, B. and Thornicroft, G. (2015) "Reversing hard won victories in the name of human rights: a critique of the General Comment on Article 12 of the UN Convention on the Rights of Persons with Disabilities." *The Lancet*, 2(9): 844–885.

Mental Welfare Commission for Scotland. (2014) "Deprivation of Liberty." Available from: http://www.mwcscot.org.uk/media/124856/mwc_deprivation_of_libertyanalysis-2.pdf.

Mental Welfare Commission for Scotland. (2016) "Supported Decision Making." Available from; http://www.mwcscot.org.uk/media/348023/mwc_sdm_draft_gp_guide_10__post_board__jw_final.pdf.

Northern Ireland Assembly: Mental Capacity Act (Northern Ireland). (2016) Available from: http://www.legislation.gov.uk/nia/2016/18/contents/enacted.

Scottish Parliament: Adults with Incapacity (Scotland) Act. (2000) Available from: http://www.legislation.gov.uk/asp/2000/4/contents.

United Kingdom Parliament: Human Rights Act. (1998) Available from: http://www.legislation.gov.uk/ukpga/1998/42/contents.

United Nations. (2006) "Convention on the Rights of Persons with Disabilities." Available from: http://www.un.org/disabilities/convention/conventionfull.shtml.

United Nations Committee on the Rights of Persons with Disabilities. (2014) "General comment No. 1 Article 12: Equal recognition before the law." Available from: https://documents-dds-ny.un.org/doc/UNDOC/GEN/G14/031/20/PDF/G1403120.pdf?OpenElement.

University of Essex: Essex Autonomy Project. (2014) "Is the MCA compliant with the UNCRPD: Briefing Papers." Available from: http://autonomy.essex.ac.uk/is-the-mca-compliant-with-the-uncrpd-briefing-papers.

University of Essex: Essex Autonomy Project. (2016) "Towards Compliance with CRPD Art. 12 in Capacity/Incapacity Legislation across the UK." Available from: http://autonomy.essex.ac.uk/uncrpd.

13 Education, training and dementia

Anna Jack-Waugh and Margaret Brown

Introduction

Dementia has a major impact on every health and social care system in the world, with accompanying economic and workforce challenges. Demographic change shows increasing numbers of people affected by dementia, and it is acknowledged that "specialist" dementia services will no longer have the capacity to meet this growing need (Alzheimer's Disease International 2016). This will affect social and health care practitioners and educational preparation is needed at all levels. Improving knowledge and skills throughout services will improve care and provide better systems of care provision (Alzheimer's Disease International 2016). In the future, it is likely that management and care currently provided by specialist mental health services will increasingly become the responsibility of primary care practitioners. The non-specialist and primary care workforce requirement for education is likely to be concerned with the diagnosis, post-diagnostic support, treatment, continuing care and end-of-life care. The role of specialist services will then focus on those groups of people with dementia who have complex needs, providing advice and training, mentoring and supervision for non-specialist practitioners.

Education and skills development for the health and social care workforce is an international concern (Collier et al. 2015). The UK, in common with the rest of the world, has a predicted rise in the incidence of people living with dementia and a decreasing pool of future practitioners and informal carers, with implications for quality of life and care (Tsaroucha et al. 2013).

With a drive to diagnose dementia earlier in the condition, health and social care staff will be in contact with people living with dementia in a range of settings (Alushi et al. 2015). In the UK, critical reports, national strategies and guidelines on dementia have emphasised the need for education to address the challenges working with older people with dementia and complex needs across all health services (Banerjee et al. 2016). Yet there has been a significant lack of research on education that will support practitioners to work with people with dementia in community settings (Elliott et al. 2012). The World Health Organization (2012) has identified that developing knowledge and skills with healthcare professionals involved in the treatment of people with dementia is a priority area. The European Parliament has called on countries across Europe to develop action plans and create common guidelines to inform the education and training of professionals caring for people with dementia.

Up to 25% of patients in acute hospitals have a form of dementia. It is frequently reported that care in hospitals can lack dignity, be frightening and increase the complexity of both physical and mental ill-health, leading to reduced discharge options and increased mortality (Boaden 2016; Royal College of Psychiatrists 2011). As most people living with dementia are older, consideration must also be given to their complex health needs (Baillie et al. 2015). There has been a consistent call for all hospital staff to be dementia aware and educated appropriately to their role (Boaden 2016). Nurses are an important group to target as they make up the largest proportion of health care professionals and work in diverse settings.

Current knowledge

Higher education and dementia

Higher education institutions have a key role to play in the provision of high-quality dementia education in academic programmes for all health and social care professionals (Collier et al. 2015). Despite this, a survey of all UK higher education institutions found that education about dementia in health and social care courses was mainly absent. In a survey of 22 higher education institutions, mental health nursing programmes ranged from three to 54 hours, in adult nursing, allied health professionals and social work programmes it was 0–6 hours (Pulsford et al. 2007). Although this study has not been repeated, specialist educators assert that this situation remains unchanged (Collier et al. 2015). In addition to the lack of pre-registration training, 95% of hospitals in England had no mandatory training in dementia for any staff (Royal College of Psychiatrists, 2011).

Box 13.1 Reflection

Consider your first experience of professional education in health or social care.
   Can you recall the dementia related content of your course?
   To what extent did this prepare you to provide care and support to people affected by dementia?

Internationally, most dementia strategies have education of the dementia workforce as a key action; in the UK, this is a priority. This has led to the development of the Curricular Standards to support Dementia Education (Richards et al. 2014). In Scotland, Promoting Excellence Knowledge and Skills Framework preceded this and has increasingly led the focus of educational provision in Scotland since it was published (Scottish Government 2011).

These UK initiatives provide a context for practitioners, educators, and policymakers. Below are excerpts that compare the Curricular Standards for Dementia Education, focussing on health practitioners and the Promoting Excellence Framework, supporting all staff working in health and social care. The development, underpinning ethos and integrative nature of them differ significantly in detail.

Box 13.2 Activity

Standards for Dementia Education:
  Access and compare the two documents below.

Department of Health, Skills for Health, and Health Education England (2015) Dementia Core Skills Education and Training Framework. http://www.skillsforhealth.org.uk/images/projects/dementia/Dementia%20Core%20Skills%20Education%20and%20Training%20Framework.pdf.

Scotland: Promoting Excellence Framework (Scottish Government 2011). http://www.gov.scot/resource/doc/350174/0117211.pdf

Consider how these two frameworks are similar or different.
How does each framework make recommendations for values based practice, preservation of human rights and person-centred practice?

There is a need for clear *and* comprehensive guidance for education, whether in single or multi-professional groups. The development of shared and detailed curricular standards could support the development of a professional and academic pathway for practitioners. This would result in a shared vision to meet the aspirations of people affected by dementia.

There is still a challenge in higher education arising from the lack of focus on dementia in professional education over many years. Teaching staff may also have lacked opportunity in the past to develop dementia expertise. Further, the demand for education in dementia is not matched by a rise in the number of educators, with dwindling workforce resources for education, reducing the provision of programmes. Education about dementia can be a tick box exercise, with a tension between simply doing it, versus doing it well (Collier et al. 2015).

Effective higher education and dementia

Pre-registration programmes are the precursor to professional practice. Failure to develop future professionals with the appropriate values, knowledge and skills to work effectively in partnership with people with dementia, will risk skills and knowledge remaining at the current level. After qualification, the lack of a consistent approach to developing the education of the professional will affect evidence-informed health and social care provision. As a result there will be little research capacity to support this.

There are significant gaps in what is understood about how effective pre-registration and post-registration dementia education is for practitioners (Hvalič-Touzery et al. 2018). There are no current studies in the UK and Europe specifically researching pre-registration programmes content on dementia (Alushi et al. 2015). Those studies that are available are from North America and highlight the need for a clear interplay between good theoretical preparation before a student attends relevant practice placements. The aim of pre-registration programmes should include improving knowledge, attitudes and communication when working with people living with dementia. Short periods of exposure to theory and practice, common in undergraduate programmes, do not work. Instead prolonged engagement over time is needed. This preparation helps students understand the specialised nature of care and management of care for the person affected by dementia (Banerjee et al. 2016).

Box 13.3 Innovations in education

In one medical programme the Time for Dementia project involved students spending time with people with dementia while carrying out:

- conversations concerning the impact of dementia and the experience of using health and social care services;
- life story work, reviewing and discussing the person life;
- a "This is Me" document with the person which is a structured approach to supporting person-centred care;
- completing a reflective practice portfolio.

The programme ended with a conference for all the people with dementia and students involved. This innovative approach was concerned with understanding the experience, lives and aspirations of the person living with dementia and learning about a human rights partnerships approach.

There are more examples of continuing professional development programmes focussed upon the care of people with dementia in general hospitals, (Banks et al. 2014; Elvish et al. 2016). However, there is concern about the quality of educational interventions surrounding content, effectiveness and methods of evaluation (Tullo et al. 2015). It is important to develop evidence-based educational approaches that clearly show evidence of effectiveness. However, even more, important is demonstrating that education is having an impact on the experience and outcomes for people with dementia in hospital.

Challenges for education in dementia

There are some areas that present a challenge for educational provision. These include education about the advanced stages of dementia within primary care and specialist dementia services. As there will be an increasing number of people living with dementia as the condition advances, then education about this period will become increasingly important. For the person with advanced dementia, quality care requires a skilled and knowledgeable workforce. This is currently in short supply across Europe (Hvalič-Touzery et al. 2018).

Box 13.4 Research into practice: The Palliare project

Palliare refers to the often extended and prolonged, advanced phase of dementia. The Dementia Palliare project has worked across seven countries between 2014 and 2016. It supports the qualified dementia workforce to deliver evidence-informed improvements for people in the advanced stage of dementia and family caring through developing educational modules and an online community of practice.

Detailed information can be sourced by following the links in the further reading section.

Preconceived ideas about dementia have led to negative stereotypes often rein-forced by the media (Riley et al. 2014). Following Kitwood (1997) who described how people with dementia were treated as separate, other and lacking in person-hood, the impact of stigma can lead to exclusion and reduce the quality of care. For people at the point of diagnosis, stigma was reported to be one of the greatest barriers to seeking help and accessing support, treatment and information (Milne 2009).

Stigma can have an impact on staff too, and many healthcare professionals hold negative views towards caring for older people with dementia (Tullo et al. 2015). Caring for people with dementia can be perceived as having low social status, requiring minimal skills and knowledge. Education has to recognise this concern and develop rights-based learning to challenge negative values and attitudes. Stigma and negative approaches are already being challenged by the increasing number of people living well with dementia, the drive to ensure dementia is evident in the education of all health and social care practitioners and the policies and directives which emphasise rights-based citizenship.

Box 13.5 Example of good practice: The Scottish experience

The Dementia Champions programme in particular creates a direct link between carers of people with dementia and the wide range of health and social care professionals who support them. This ensures the views and experiences of carers inform practice and professional development.

National Dementia Carers Action Network (NDCAN, with permission)

Scotland's approach began with the Charter of Rights for People with Dementia and their Carers (Alzheimer Scotland 2009), which combats institutional and stigmatised care. Scotland's first National Dementia Strategy (Scottish Government 2010) inspired the Promoting Excellence Framework (PEF) of knowledge and skills relevant for all staff working with people with dementia in health and social services (Scottish Government 2011). This is based on a human rights-based approach to promote practice underpinned by positive values.

The Framework includes four levels of knowledge and skills (Dementia Informed Practice, Dementia Skilled Practice, Enhanced Dementia Practice and Expertise in Dementia Practice) ranging from baseline skills for the entire workforce through to expert specialist roles. A recent report highlighted that all Scottish Universities are providing undergraduate nursing or social work degree programmes are working towards all students achieving "Skilled Level". A delivery plan is supported by integrated online learning areas, learning resources and a range of face-to-face events delivered across all sectors. There are key roles developed to support the delivery plan in practice, including Dementia Ambassadors, Dementia Champions, Dementia Nurse and Allied Health Professional Consultants. While this example of Scotland's approach to educating the dementia workforce requires further research and evaluation, it may provide long-term impact on improving coordination between educators and trainers in different settings.

Inter-professional education (IPE), where two or more professions learn with and from each other is favoured as a method for developing a collaborative practice. If the changing approach to working with people with dementia discussed earlier becomes a reality, IPE will be essential. However, a systematic review highlighted that the body of evidence examining IPE for staff around dementia was of a weak methodological quality (Jackson et al. 2016). Despite the lack of evidence so far, IPE will be an essential model for the development of the current and future workforces and the development of care for people with dementia. Robust research into effectiveness and methods of IPE focussing on dementia education is needed.

Practice recommendations

In line with international social policy, all professionals will need to be competent and confident to work with people with dementia irrespective of which service they work in. The potential positive impact of IPE on the outcomes for people with dementia and their families should be considered alongside the changes in the delivery of care pathways. To do this, higher education institutions have an important role to play in equipping health and social care practitioners with knowledge and skills for all those affected throughout the dementia journey. This should include the creation of enriched care environments for those affected by living for many months or years with advanced dementia.

A firm foundation should be developed in the person's first professional preparation. HEIs have an opportunity to provide contemporary, stimulating and evidence-based education. This will support developing professionals and help them to acknowledge and challenge preconceptions. Educational interventions will include consideration of the impact of stigma and a human rights-based approach to developing positive professional values. Further research into pre-registration education should evaluate teaching methods and the interplay between theory and practice. Part of this is about providing the opportunity to develop longer-term relationships between students and people living with dementia, their family and supporters.

Education for practitioners should have a shared vision of essential content and learning approaches, achieved by the use of curricula standards or knowledge and skills frameworks. Further research is required into how curricula are translated across education and the impact this has on improving the standards of direct patient care. Research is needed into the impact of education for hospital and inter-professional groups of practitioners and there is a lack of evidence about the impact of education on those who care for the person with dementia living at home.

A consistent approach to educational philosophy, content and structure could build capacity for excellent knowledge and skills in dementia care for both practitioners and academics. This consistency will lead to the provision of evidence informed practice by an appropriately knowledgeable and skilled workforce working with people living with dementia, now and in the future.

References

Alushi, L., Hammond, J. A. and Wood, J. H. (2015) "Evaluation of dementia education programs for pre-registration healthcare students – A review of the literature." *Nurse Education Today*, 35(9): 992–998.

Alzheimer's Disease International. (2016) "World Alzheimer Report 2016 – Improving healthcare for people living with dementia: coverage, quality and costs now and in the future." London:

A.s.D. International. Available from: https://www.alz.co.uk/research/WorldAlzheimerRep ort2016.pdf.

Alzheimer Scotland. (2009) "Charter of Rights for People with Dementia and their Carers." Available from: http://www.alzscot.org/assets/0000/2678/Charter_of_Rights.pdf.

Baillie, L., Merritt, J., Cox, J. and Crichton, N. (2015) "Confidence and expectations about caring for older people with dementia: a cross-sectional survey of student nurses." *Educational Gerontology*, 41(9): 670–682.

Banerjee, S., Farina, N., Daley, S., Grosvenor, W., Hughes, L., Hebditch, M., Mackrell, S., Nilforooshan, R., Wyatt, C., Vries, K., Haq, I. and Wright, J. (2016) "How do we enhance undergraduate healthcare education in dementia? A review of the role of innovative approaches and development of the time for dementia programme." *International Journal of Geriatric Psychiatry*, 32(1): 68–75.

Banks, P., Waugh, A., Henderson, J., Sharp, B., Brown, M., Oliver, J. and Marland, G. (2014) "Enriching the care of patients with dementia in acute settings? The Dementia Champions Programme in Scotland. " *Dementia* 3(6): 717–736. Available from: https://doi.org/10.1177/ 1471301213485084.

Boaden, A. (2016) "Alzheimer Society Fix Dementia Care: Hospitals." London: Alzheimer Society. Available from: https://www.alzheimers.org.uk/site/scripts/download_info.php?fileID=2907.

Brown, M., Waugh, A., Sharp, B., Duffy, R. and MacRae, R. (2018) "What are dementia champions and why do we need them?" *Dementia*, 17. Available from: http://journals.sagepub. com/doi/abs/10.1177/1471301217743413.

Collier, E., Knifton, C. and Surr, C. (2015) "Dementia education in Higher Education Institutions." *Nurse Education Today*, 35(6): 731–732.

Department of Health, Skills for Health, and Health Education England. (2015) "Dementia Core Skills Education and Training Framework." Available from: http://www.skillsforhealth. org.uk/images/projects/dementia/Dementia%20Core%20Skills%20Education%20and%20Tra ining%20Framework.pdf.

Elliott, K.-E. J., Scott, J. L., Stirling, C., Martin, A. J. and Robinson, A. (2012) "Building capacity and resilience in the dementia care workforce: a systematic review of interventions targeting worker and organizational outcomes." *International Psychogeriatrics*, 24(6): 882.

Elvish, R., Burrow, S., Cawley, R., Harney, K., Pilling, M., Gregory, J. and Keady, J. (2016) "'Getting to Know Me': The second phase roll-out of a staff training programme for sup- porting people with dementia in general hospitals." *Dementia*, 17(1): 96–109. Available from: https://doi.org/10.1177/1471301216634926.

Hvalič-Touzery, S., Skela-Savič, B., Macrae, R., Jack-Waugh, A., Tolson, D., Hellström, A., de Abreu, W. and Pesjak, K. (2018) "The provision of accredited higher education on dementia in six European countries: An exploratory study." *Nurse Education Today*, 60: 161–169.

Jackson, M., Pelone, F., Reeves, S., Hassenkamp, A. M., Emery, C., Titmarsh, K. and Green- wood, N. (2016) "Interprofessional education in the care of people diagnosed with dementia and their carers: a systematic review." *BMJ Open*, 6: e010948. doi:10.1136/bmjopen-2015-010948.

Kitwood, T.M. (1997) *Dementia Reconsidered: The Person Comes First*. London: Open Uni- versity Press.

Milne, A.(2010) "The 'D' word: Reflections on the relationship between stigma, discrimination and dementia." *Journal of Mental Health*, 19(3): 227–233. doi:10.3109/09638231003728166.

Pulsford, D., Hope, K. and Thompson, R. (2007) "Higher education provision for professionals working with people with dementia: a scoping exercise." *Nurse Education Today*, 27(1): 5–13.

Riley, R.J., Burgener, S. and Buckwalter, K.C. (2014) "Anxiety and stigma in dementia: a threat to aging in place." *The Nursing Clinics of North America*, 49(2): 213–231.

Royal College of Psychiatrists. (2011) "Report of the National Audit of Dementia Care in Gen- eral Hospitals NATIONAL REPORT." Available from: https://www.rcpsych.ac.uk/pdf/ NATIONAL%20REPORT%20-%20Full%20Report%201201122.pdf.

Scottish Government. (2010) "Scotland's National Dementia Strategy." Available from: http://www.gov.scot/Resource/Doc/324377/0104420.pdf .

Scottish Government. (2011) "Promoting Excellence: A framework for all health and social services staff working with people with dementia, their families and carers." Available from: http://www.gov.scot/resource/doc/350174/0117211.pdf.

Tsaroucha, A., Benbow, S. M., Kingston, P. and Le Mesurier, N. (2013) "Dementia skills for all: A core competency framework for the workforce in the United Kingdom." *Dementia: The International Journal of Social Research and Practice*, 12(1): 29–44.

Tullo, E., Khoo, T.K. and Teodorczuk, A. (2015) "Preparing to meet the needs of an ageing population – A challenge to medical educators globally." *Medical Teacher*, 37(2): 105–107.

World Health Organization. (2012) "Dementia – A public health priority." Geneva: WHO Press. Available from: https://extranet.who.int/agefriendlyworld/wp-content/uploads/2014/06/WHO-Dementia-English.pdf.

Further reading

Full details of the Palliare project can be found here: http://ec.europa.eu/programmes/proxy/alfresco-webscripts/api/node/content/workspace/SpacesStore/1d515ad0-7159-4095-a4d3-6d4748c725d4/App%2022%20Brochure_ING_final.pdf.

The Palliare Best Practice in Advanced Dementia Care is available here: http://ec.europa.eu/programmes/proxy/alfresco-webscripts/api/node/content/workspace/SpacesStore/5943dcc2-30fe-4dc3-8eb0-2bb32bc14354/app%208%20Dementia%20Palliare%20BPS%202016%20Print.pdf.

Surr, C.A., Gates, C., Irving, D., Oyebode, J., Smith, S.J., Parveen, S., Drury, M. and Dennison, A. (2017) "Effective dementia education and training for the health and social care workforce: a systematic review of the literature." *Review of Educational Research*, 87(5): 966–1002.

Tolson, D., Fleming, A., Hanson, E., Abreu, W., Crespo, M. L., Macrae, R., Jackson, G., Hvalič-Touzery, S., Routasalo, P. and Holmerová, I. (2016) "Achieving prudent dementia care (Palliare): an international policy and practice imperative." *International Journal of Integrated Care*, 16(4): 1–11.

14 The impact of later life illnesses on people living with dementia

F. J. Raymond Duffy

Introduction

People are living longer and the population is ageing. One of the consequences of this as we know has been that more people are developing dementias. However dementia is not the only long-term condition that may develop as we age. There are many other long-term conditions (or chronic diseases) that are on the increase within the wider population as a result of population ageing, such as diabetes, chronic obstructive pulmonary disease, arthritis and hypertension. People with dementia are not immune to these other conditions, in fact Barnett et al. (2012) indicate that seven in ten people who are living with dementia are also living with another concurrent medical condition and often more than one (See Figure 9.1).

Barnett et al. (2012) indicated that:

- 41% had high blood pressure
- 32% had depression
- 27% had heart disease
- 18% have had a stroke or transient ischemic attack
- 13% had diabetes

The relationship between dementia and comorbidities can be complex and variable. There are for example, many pre-existing medical conditions that increase the risk of dementia developing including:

- high blood pressure
- type 2 diabetes
- stroke
- Parkinson's disease

Certain comorbid medical conditions may also exacerbate the progression of dementia, for example, cognitive decline may be accelerated in older people with Stroke (Savva and Stephan 2010) and Type 2 diabetes (Biessels et al. 2006).

So there may be a dynamic for some people where failing to deal with their long term conditions appropriately may worsen or quicken the progress of their dementia. The presence of dementia may also mean people are less likely to receive the same help to manage and treat comorbidities than people without dementia (Scrutton and Bricanti 2016). As a result, this group suffer a faster decline in daily functioning, a reduced quality of life, and die earlier than people who have the same comorbidities, but do not have dementia.

They are also trying to negotiate their way through health and social care systems that do not always have the capacity to manage the complexity of their conditions and their day-to-day lives (Fox et al. 2014).

This chapter will look at the commonest comorbidities that may arise as we age. It will highlight the consequences of comorbidity and will look at the impact and challenges that these cause to the person living with dementia and their carers. It will consider what we can do to improve the way that health and social care professionals manage comorbidity so that they can make life for the person living with dementia and their carers a bit easier.

Common comorbidities

There are some common comorbidities amongst people with dementia. Poblador-Plou et al. (2014) found that hypertension and diabetes were the comorbidities most frequently found in older people with dementia. Although, their analysis revealed that both these conditions are common in older people in general they also identified 12 conditions that appear to be "significantly associated" with dementia: Parkinson's disease, congestive heart failure, cerebrovascular disease, anaemia, cardiac arrhythmia, chronic skin ulcers, osteoporosis, thyroid disease, retinal disorders, prostatic hypertrophy, insomnia and anxiety/neurosis. Other international studies (Löppönen et al. 2004; Bauer et al. 2013) have shown comparable results.

For most of these comorbidities, a plausible pathophysiological explanation can be found. Some could be considered as risk factors (cerebrovascular disease), others as complications (skin ulcers), and others are coincidental comorbidities (osteoporosis). However, while there may be some commonalities in the comorbidities it is important to remember that there are a number of different dementias. Any common profile reflects the situation of people with Alzheimer's disease because that is the commonest form of dementia. However, we need to bear in mind that people who have Lewy Body Dementia for example, have been found to have worse comorbidity profiles, with a higher occurrence of depression, stroke and migraine, compared with patients with Alzheimer's disease (Fereshtehnejad 2014).

A common problem highlighted by Scrutton and Brancati (2016) is that people with dementia often have atypical presentations. Changes in health status in people with dementia often present as increased confusion, falls, loss of appetite or dehydration making the connection between the symptoms and an underlying comorbidity less obvious. For example, Freidenberg (2013) found that patients with dementia were less likely to have clear hypotension symptoms like dizziness, and instead presented with symptoms such as mental fluctuations, confusion, drowsiness and falls. This may lead to health professionals and carers interpreting these problems as worsening dementia and so neglecting other conditions as a potential cause. This not only delays diagnosis but it also prevents specific treatments that could potentially improve the person's daily functioning and quality of life. On many occasions situations arise where health and social care services treat multiple illnesses in isolation from one another. This treatment of comorbidities within separate silos of specialism continues to be a barrier to diagnosis, management and support (Barnett et al. 2012). This has led to the All Party Parliamentary Group on Dementia (APPGD) (2016) emphasising the need for health and social care services to be organised in ways that treat multi-morbidity as the norm, rather than the exception.

The impact and challenge of comorbidities

With dementia affecting memory, language, problem-solving and communication, self-managing the symptoms and treatment regimens associated with other long-term conditions becomes increasingly difficult. When we consider other more expected aspects of growing older, for example deterioration in eyesight or hearing and physical losses such as muscle weakness and reduced grip strength it is clear that for many people with dementia self-management can quickly become poor management. For example, someone managing diabetes must carry out self-testing and administer insulin at certain times of the day. As a result of dementia, their ability to carry out this task will deteriorate as their memory and cognition worsen, with responsibility eventually often falling to a carer (see Box 14.1: Voices of carers).

Box 14.1 Voices of carers

The APPG (2016) recognised that as people living with dementia progressed through their illness carers end up taking significant responsibility for supporting people with increasingly complex needs, sometimes even going as far as trying to co-ordinate care. Carers reported that commonly healthcare workers only focused on the specific condition being dealt with and it fell on them to ensure the whole picture was looked at. Carers and people living with dementia were concerned about the number of agencies dealing with them, who all expected them to engage with them, or attend appointments etc., and they were having to choose between them in order to manage. Regarding the complexity of care delivery, this extract from a Carers blog is quite revealing. This entry is called *"I'm exhausted from being a Care Partner"*. The carer is discussing his wife who has a history of vascular illness and mixed dementia the carer says:

> This evening.... She is very frightened and is seeking continual reassurance but wanting to tell me things in case she forgets them. When I look back I made many mistakes last night ...exhausted Care Partners all struggle to make the right interventions!
>
> Fortunately, our social worker will be here at 11 am this morning for a routine call. The social worker's assessment is that...my wife... has capacity... but unfortunately, all she has to go on is what she sees, and hears, in her occasional visits. It's difficult for anyone to see... (how distressed she becomes)... her functional capacity and "out of character" behaviours are kept well-hidden from professional staff.
>
> My priority is to help (her) settle down, and re-establish harmony. I think it is an opportune moment to seek a Case Conference to consider my wife's presentation, and my responses as a Care Partner. In the interim period there are a number of measures that need to be taken:
> - To check for UTI or other type of infection.
> - To review the nature and frequency of the carer sitting service

- To encourage (my wife) to take more exercise.
- To try to entice (my wife) into new activities: particularly in the evenings.
- To organise carer respite, possibly overnight, ASAP.
- To reduce the pain in my own limbs, and left shoulder.

Continued poor management of a health condition can lead to someone falling seriously ill, resulting in an emergency hospital admission. It can also mean that the progression of other long-term conditions is more rapid when compared to the progress of the illness in those without dementia (Bunn et al. 2016; Snowden et al. 2017).

Added to this, dementia itself will increase the risk of people receiving poor care for their other conditions. Fox et al. (2014) point out that people living with dementia and comorbidities are less likely to receive the equivalent level of care for similar conditions than people living without dementia due to delays in the recognition of new or exacerbating symptoms. Studies have found for example that people with dementia were less likely to receive monitoring for diabetes related problems (Feil et al. 2011), had reduced access to treatment, such as intravenous thrombolysis for stroke (Bunn et al. 2016), surgery for cataracts and treatment for age-related macular degeneration (Bartlett and McKeefry 2009) and evidence that pain experienced by people with dementia and arthritis was also undertreated (Balfour and O'Rourke 2003).

This situation is also aggravated because people with dementia may not notice and may not report relevant symptoms. They are also more likely to struggle to attend regular appointments and be much more reliant on carers to facilitate and manage their contacts and appointments with health and social care services.

Clinicians may be more reluctant to investigate and treat people with dementia either because of the difficulties involved in securing patient cooperation, or because treatments are considered inappropriate for older patients with multi-morbidity. In addition, if the dementia is symptomatic because the person is demonstrating behavioural and psychological symptoms associated with dementia, then dementia may become the focus of clinical contacts and detract from the management of other chronic conditions such as diabetes (Piette and Kerr 2006).

The impact on carers

As a person's dementia progresses, it is their carers who often end up having significant responsibility in helping the person deal with their increasingly complex needs. Carers may do everything from providing meals to administering medicine, even extending to co-ordinating someone's care. Often the carers find themselves struggling because they don't have enough information about all the health conditions their loved ones are affected by or how these conditions may interact or interrelate with one another. In addition, carers are not fully informed on how to manage these conditions collectively or where to turn for care and support. This can lead to carers taking on too much often unknowingly and then burning out or feeling helpless to prevent crises that could have been averted if they had been able to access more professional help (APPGD 2016).

Carers have also expressed concerns that they felt that they received inadequate support in planning the person with dementia's care and that their contribution to managing that care was not always recognised. Furthermore they felt that they were often excluded from decision making despite the important role they play in ensuring care continuity (Fiel et al. 2011).

The financial implications of the mismanagement of people with dementia who have a comorbid illness are staggering. Research by the International Longevity Centre – UK (ILC) found that people with dementia are less likely to have cases of depression, diabetes or urinary tract infections diagnosed. Those that do get a diagnosis are less likely to receive the same help to manage and treat them, so a consequence is that the person's dementia progresses more quickly raising their health and social care costs. The ILC-UK estimate the combined cost for mismanagement of dementia with depression, diabetes or urinary tract infections alone was at least £994.4 million in 2016 in the UK alone (Scrutton and Brancanti 2016).

Where can we do things better?

In the long run the most significant thing that can be done to reduce the occurrence of these issues amongst people living with dementia, is to act to avoid the development of the chronic diseases responsible for most comorbidity. As the World Health Organisation (WHO) (2008) point out, inexpensive and cost-effective interventions can prevent 80% of heart disease, stroke, type 2 diabetes and 40% of cancers. There is strong scientific evidence supporting the fact that a healthy diet and sufficient physical activity are key elements in the prevention of long-term conditions and their risk factors. There is also evidence that careful management of diet, exercise, not smoking and the avoidance of depression from middle age are particularly important in decreasing someone's likelihood of developing dementia and related comorbidities (Norton et al. 2014). Moreover, attention to alcohol intake and sleep hygiene in midlife also has known health benefits. The following are also being explored as potential routes to avoiding dementia and other comorbidities: passive smoking, reducing exposure to excessive noise, cognitive stimulation, the effect of participation in social activities, head injury prevention and attention to reproductive health (Rooney 2014).

This emphasis on focussing and improving health promotion in midlife however will have little impact on those who have or who are developing dementia currently. Perhaps the most significant step that could be taken is to address concerns that healthcare professionals have about the lack of guidance available around prescribing safely and effectively to older people with multiple morbidities (APPGD 2016). In 2016, the National Institute for Health and Care Excellence (NICE) released their first guideline on the clinical assessment and management of multimorbidity (NICE 2016). While the focus of this guidance is on frailty, a large number of people with dementia are frail and may benefit from this as the goal of the guidance is to reduce the treatment burden and optimise care and support by encouraging people with multimorbidities and their families to clarify what is important to them, including their personal goals, values and priorities.

However although the guideline states that there is a need to identify an accurate list of a person's current medicines and then compare that with what the person actually uses, and recommends review as a consequence, there is no recognised national or international guidance on polypharmacy. There is even less guidance to address how to tackle polypharmacy in people living with dementia and multiple long-term conditions.

Finally very little is known about how family carers can best be supported to deal with their loved one who has both dementia and multiple long-term conditions, or how health care services should adapt to address their particular needs (Scrutton and Brancati 2016; APPGD 2016).

Practice recommendations

Firstly, there are a number of components to what is recognised as good personalised health and social care that would be very effective in ensuring that people with dementia who have other long-term conditions receive the support they need from health and social care services. These components are access to good quality information, the utilisation of a comprehensive care plan that is updated regularly, consistent multi-disciplinary assessment that includes regular reviews of care and support and someone who will act as a care co-ordinator (Alzheimer Scotland 2012). Providing care that delivers these components will help the person and their family achieve the integrated care and support they need from health and social care services. This will enable them to self-manage their conditions more effectively. This will both reduce the risk of admission and has the potential to reduce care costs. Whilst the importance of providing personalised community care is widely recognised in public policy (e.g. The Care Act 2014) many people with dementia and comorbidities struggle to get this level of care in practice (APPGD 2016).

The management of multiple long-term conditions is the principle challenge for health and social care services this century (WHO 2013). As we have seen poor medication management and a lack of support to aid self-management and management by carers means that urgent action is needed if we are to see this group of people better sustained. A lot of the action required is not just needed for this particular group of people with multiple long-term conditions but is required to ensure that all health and social care services are equipped to support people with multiple comorbidities to live contented lives.

Without a radical change in focus and priority, we risk consigning many more people to substandard care and a poor quality of life (Bunn et al. 2016, Scrutton and Bracanti 2016; WHO 2013). Optimizing the treatment of co-morbidities in people with dementia has the potential to improve their early prognosis meaning that managing comorbidity may offer an opportunity to prevent some of the complications of dementia, such as falls and infection, which could further reduce care costs (Scrutton and Bracanti 2016).

Partly because of the difficulties that health and social care professionals have in assessing and monitoring comorbidities in this group and in response to the difficulties posed to people presenting with dementia and their carers having to deal with getting to separate reviews for each long-term condition, the APPGD (2016) recommended that people known to have dementia and comorbidities should have a minimum of one comprehensive, holistic review of their health per year. This should initially be led by a GP, and draw on other health and social care professionals as required. This should be reflected in an update of all aspects of a person's care plan, from medication to social care support. This would be a good starting point for re-evaluating the way care is delivered to people living with dementia and other chronic illnesses (see Box 14.2 Tips for good practice, which summarises some key points).

Box 14.2 Tips for good practice

- People living with dementia and their carers should have access to good quality information about comorbid illnesses as well as dementia.
- A holistic multidisciplinary personalised care plan should be in place that identifies a person responsible for care co-ordination.
- The support offered to carers is key to ensuring that people living with both dementia and other co-morbid illness/es continue to manage their healthcare within their own community and avoid costly admission to healthcare facilities.
- A single comprehensive annual review (at a minimum) carried out and co-ordinated by a primary healthcare practitioner (GP) with access to a wider team should be a compulsory component of all people living with dementia and other long-term illnesses care.

There is however also a pressing issue in this area, which is just how little we know about the human response to dealing with dementia while having other long-term conditions.

Currently there is a lack of research on the experiences of people with dementia and their family carers on living and dying with dementia and comorbid conditions. Although health care professionals acknowledge the vital role that family carers play in managing the healthcare conditions of people living with dementia, facilitating both continuity of care and the person's access to care, this recognition does not translate into their routine involvement in appointments or decision-making about the person they are caring for. There is work required to identify how people with dementia deal with their comorbidities and how best they could be supported. Even more work is needed to understand the views and roles of carers so that their position is both better understood and sustained. The APPGD (2016) found examples of good practice across the UK but as they state, these tended to be about the behaviour of individual practitioners rather than system-based, evidence-based approaches to management. In fact they criticised current systems which may be unintentionally blocking access to care for people living with dementia and their families by failing to act in a holistic and integrated manner, often leaving people to pick and choose the interventions to engage with on very little information (APPGD 2016; Bunn et al. 2014) (see Box 14.3 Good practice example, Oxleas Advanced Dementia Service)

Box 14.3 Good practice example

Oxleas Advanced Dementia Service provides holistic and palliative care at home for people with advanced dementia. The service is constructed so that a core team of old-age psychiatrists, mental health and community staff work with GPs, secondary care and social services to support family and/or carers in providing ongoing and palliative care to people living with dementia. The service works with family and carers to prevent hospital or care home admission, navigating through the complex health and social care system as people's needs and their entitlements to support change. The key lessons from their work are as follows:

- A focus on building resilience amongst carers.
- They accept referrals form a wide range of healthcare professionals.

- They identify suitable people for the service via the strong links they have with both community and community mental healthcare teams.
- The development of a holistic assessment and resulting personalised care plan which includes a plan for dealing with potential crises.
- Care co-ordination of care via a primary contact person.
- Rapid access to advice and support from a multidisciplinary team via the care co-ordinator.

Their approach to the co-ordinated care of complex people living with dementia was the subject of an in-depth study carried out by the King's Fund in 2013. Details about their Care process and how the service is organised can be found at: https://www.kingsfund.org.uk/publications/oxleas-advanced-dementia-service.

While little may be known about the reality of the situation for people living with dementia and their carers it could be argued that even less is known about healthcare providers' experiences of managing people living with dementia and comorbid health conditions and how the presence of dementia influences their decisions and the care that people living with dementia actually receive.

Future work needs to focus on the development and evaluation of interventions to improve continuity of care and access to services for people living with dementia and other comorbidities. These studies should focus on how dementia and other significant cognitive impairments influence care provision and decisions to hospitalise which often have detrimental effect on the person and significantly increase the cost of care, particularly since in-hospital complications and re-admission are both commonplace (LoGiudice et al.. 2016).

Finally, there are a number of disease specific interactions that require further exploration. The interaction and impact of having a dementia and cardiovascular disease, stroke or diabetes and potentially combinations of all 4 stand out as requiring further study as combinations of two or more are commonplace and poor management may reduce life expectancy. The interaction of dementia with chronic pain, depression and falls has also been suggested as key comorbidities that we need to understand better. In future research it is important that people with dementia are included in the debate about the management of their comorbidities. They also need to be included in more of the studies and trials that focus on age-related comorbidity (Bunn et al. 2014).

Box 14.4 Reflective questions

What are you doing to prevent yourself from developing a long-term illness in the future, including reducing your risk of dementia? What will you tell your family and friends to do?

Presented with a person who has dementia and one of the other common co-morbidities listed in the section called "Common Comorbidities", how would you go about assessing their health and social care needs? Drawing on the expertise of the team that you work with or the circumstances that you are in, who else might you need to involve?

References

All-Party Parliamentary Group on Dementia (APPGD). (2016) *Dementia rarely travels alone: Living with dementia and other conditions.* London: Alzheimer's Society.

Alzheimer Scotland. (2012) *Delivering Integrated Dementia Care: The 8 Pillars Model of Community Support.* Edinburgh: Alzheimer Scotland. Available from: http://www.alzscot.org/assets/0000/4613/FULL_REPORT_8_Pillars_Model_of_Community_Support.pdf.

Balfour, J. and O'Rourke, N. (2003) "Older adults with Alzheimer disease, comorbid arthritis and prescription of psychotropic medications." *Pain*, 8: 198–204.

Barnett, K., Mercer, S.W., Norbury, M., Watt, G., Wyke, S. and Guthrie, B. (2012) "Epidemiology of multimorbidity and implications for health care, research, and medical education: a cross-sectional study." *The Lancet*, 380(9836): 37–43.

Bartlett, D. and McKeefry, R. (2009) "People with dementia and sight loss: a scoping study of models of care." *Research Findings*, 25. Thomas Pocklington Trust. Available from: http://pocklington-trust.org.uk/wp-content/uploads/2016/02/Dementia-care-found-lacking.pdf.

Biessels, G.J., Staekenborg, S., Brunner, E., Brayne, C. and Scheltens, P. (2006) "Risk of dementia in diabetes mellitus: a systematic review." *Lancet Neurology*, 5: 64–74.

Bauer, K., Schwarzkopf, L., Graessel, E. and Holle, R. (2014) "A claims data-based comparison of comorbidity in individuals with and without dementia." *BMC geriatrics*, 14(1): 10. Available from: http://www.biomedcentral.com/1471-2318/14/10.

Bunn, F., Burn, A.M., Goodman, C., Rait, G., Norton, S., Robinson, L., Schoeman, J. and Brayne, C. (2014) "Comorbidity and dementia: a scoping review of the literature." *BMC Medicine*, 12(1): 192. Available from: http://www.biomedcentral.com/1741-7015/12/192.

Bunn, F., Burn A-M., GoodmanC., Robinson, L., Rait, G., Norton, S., Bennett, H., Poole, M., Schoeman, J. and Brayne, C. (2016) "Comorbidity and dementia: a mixed-method study on improving health care for people with dementia (CoDem)." *Health Services and Delivery Research*, 4(8). doi:10.3310/hsdr04080.

Feil, D.G., Lukman, R., Simon, B., Walston, A. and Vickrey, B. (2011) "Impact of dementia on caring for patients' diabetes." *Aging and Mental Health*, 15: 894–903.

Fereshtehnejad, S-M. (2014) "Comorbidity profile in dementia with Lewy bodies versus Alzheimer's disease: a linkage study between the Swedish Dementia Registry and the Swedish National Patient Registry." *Alzheimer's Research & Therapy*, 6: 65. Available at: http://alzres.com/content/6/5/65.

Fox, C., Smith, T., Maidment, I., Hebding, J., Madzima, T., Cheater, F., Cross, J., Poland, F., White, J. and Young, J. (2014) "The importance of detecting and managing comorbidities in people with dementia." *Age and Ageing*, 43: 741–743. doi:10.1093/ageing/afu101.

Freidenberg, D.L. (2013) "Orthostatic hypotension in patients with dementia: clinical features and response to treatment." *Cognitive Behavioural Neurology*, 3: 105–120. Available from: http://www.ncbi.nlm.nih.gov/pubmed/24077570.

LoGiudice, D., Tropea, J., Brand, C.A., Gorelik, A. and Liew, D. (2016) "Hospitalised older people with dementia and delirium: More readmissions and in-hospital complications, greater length of stay and associated health care costs." *Alzheimer and Dementia*, 12(7), Supplement: 579.

Löppönen, M.K., Isoaho, R.E., Räihä, I.J., Vahlberg, T.J., Loikas, S.M., Takala, T.I., Puolijoki, H., Irjala, K.M. and Kivelä, S.L. (2004) "Undiagnosed diseases in patients with dementia–a potential target group for intervention." *Dementia and Geriatric Cognitive Disorders*, 18: 321–329. Available from: http://www.karger.com/Article/Pdf/80126.

National Institute for Health and Care Excellence (NICE). (2016) "NICE guideline 56: Multimorbidity: clinical assessment and management." Available from: https://www.nice.org.uk/guidance/ng56.

Norton, S., Matthews, F.E., Barnes, D.E., Yaffe, K. and Brayne, C. (2014) "Potential for primary prevention of Alzheimer's disease: an analysis of population-based data." *The Lancet Neurology*, 13(8): 788–794.

Poblador-Plou, B., Calderón-Larrañaga, A., Marta-Moreno, J., Hancco-Saavedra, J., Sicras-Mainar, A., Soljak, M. and Prados-Torres, A. (2014) "Comorbidity of dementia: a cross-sectional study of primary care older patients." *BMC psychiatry*, 14(1): 84. Available from: http://www.biomedcentral.com/1471-244X/14/84.

Piette, J.D. and Kerr, E.A. (2006) "The impact of comorbid chronic conditions on diabetes care." *Diabetes Care*, 29: 725–731.

Rooney, R. (2014) "Preventing dementia: how lifestyle in midlife affects risk." *Current Opinion in Psychiatry*, 27(2): 149–157.

Savva, G.M. and Stephan, B.C. (2010) "Alzheimer's Society Vascular Dementia Systematic Review Group: Epidemiological studies of the effect of stroke on incident dementia: a systematic review." *Stroke*, 2(41): e41–e46.

Scrutton, J. and Brancati, C.U. (2016) *Dementia and comorbidities – ensuring parity of care.* London: The International Longevity Centre – UK (ILC-UK).

Snowden, M.B., Steinman, L.E., Bryant, L.L., Cherrier, M.M., Greenlund, K.J., Leith, K.H., Levy, C., Logsdon, R.G., Copeland, C., Vogel, M. and Anderson, L.A. (2017) "Dementia and co-occurring chronic conditions: a systematic literature review to identify what is known and where are the gaps in the evidence?" *International Journal of Geriatric Psychiatry*, 32: 357–371.

World Health Organization. (2008) *WHO global strategy on diet, physical activity and health: a framework to monitor and evaluate implementation.* Geneva: WHO Press. Available from: http://www.who.int/dietphysicalactivity/DPASindicators/en/.

World Health Organization. (2013) *Global Action Plan for the Prevention and Control of NCDs 2013–2020.* Geneva: WHO Press. Available from: http://www.who.int/nmh/events/ncd_action_plan/en/.

Further reading

Bunn, F., Burn, A-M., Goodman, C., Robinson, L., Rait, G., Norton, S., Bennett, H., Poole, M., Schoeman, J., Brayne, C. (2016) "Comorbidity and dementia: a mixed-method study on improving health care for people with dementia (CoDem)." *Health Services and Delivery Research*, 4(8). doi:10.3310/hsdr04080.

"Improving healthcare for people with dementia and comorbidity." (2016). Available from: https://www.youtube.com/watch?v=jWUXaaL6Arc.

Part III
Specific issues in dementia care

15 Caring interventions

Debbie Tolson and Bryan Mitchell

Introduction

Managing life with dementia involves the individual and others adapting and responding to progressive dementia related changes centred on impairment of cognitive functions, most notably memory. As many aspects of life and social interaction depend upon cognitive functions it is important that caring and enabling interventions and approaches are provided and that practitioners and family carers understand the range of helpful enabling interventions and activities that can be provided in the family home and within any care environment. These interventions include those requiring expert practitioner knowledge and skills, to more informal social interventions that can be provided by volunteers or family members to give a sense of companionship and enjoyable social stimulation. If we take a bio-psycho-social model of dementia (Spector and Orrell 2010) then the choice of caring and enabling interventions is broad and selection will depend on the person's condition and clinical needs, emotional well-being, spirituality, their preferences and the circumstances in which they are living and the desired outcome of the intervention. As a rule of thumb interventions with therapeutic intentions should be provided by an appropriately qualified and equipped practitioner using dementia sensitive approaches. It is also wise for everyone involved in the delivery of interventions including meaningful activities such as creative arts to be dementia aware and receive training in working with people with dementia.

For example, cognitive stimulation therapies that aim to enhance cognitive and social functioning using a range of techniques to orientate the person to skills they need to live and function, should be provided by skilled and expert practitioners. Reminiscence therapy that also provides a form of cognitive stimulation requires professional knowledge, but more informal reminiscence activities that are purposeful and affirming, providing enjoyment and companionship are easily undertaken by family and friends. Passive art-based activities offer opportunity for entertainment whilst active art-based interventions offer opportunity for imaginative expression and creation. Figure 15.1 includes examples of caring interventions that are described in the practice or research literature. It is important when selecting caring interventions that you explore the evidence based for their use and avoid approaches that are demeaning or of unknown benefit.

To assist you in your selection of caring interventions we briefly explore the "outcomes" that practitioners and researchers might use to measure the impact of an intervention, moving to the more personal outcomes and experiences important to the individual and or relatives. We discuss one of the most popular types of interventions used within dementia care, namely reminiscence and introduce new work on the use of complementary therapy within advanced dementia care.

Caring Intervention	Description
Reminiscence	Activities that stimulate a person or groups to talk about the past.
Music Therapy	Music based interventions that may involve playing instruments, listening or singing.
Dementia Dogs	Dogs trained to support people with dementia to perform selected tasks, to provide companionship and comfort.
Doll Therapy	Lifelike baby dolls designed to evoke positive nurturing responses linked to memories of parenthood.
Playlist for Life	Personalised set of favourite songs and pieces of music.

Figure 15.1 Examples of caring interventions used within dementia care

From measures to personal outcomes

The quest for evidence informed dementia practice and care has naturally followed the changing views on the nature and diversity of evidence for practice (see Chapter 22).

Box 15.1 Reflective questions

- What caring interventions are available for people with early onset dementia?
- How do cultural and gender aspects influence preferences for caring interventions and how feasible is it in practice to deliver caring interventions that embrace diversity?

Dementia is caused by diseases that damage the brain, accordingly it is important to consider how enabling interventions and purposeful activities influence and improve dementia related symptoms.

As discussed in Chapter 16, neuropsychiatric symptoms are common in dementia and there is growing consensus in the literature that scores on specific symptom clusters such as measures of affect, apathy and so on may be more meaningful than overall scores. The dementia symptoms and behaviours that are most important to the interventions explored in this chapter include cognitive performance and memory, communication, agitation, apathy, sleep pattern, eating and drinking. In the UK one of the most popular scales for clinical purposes and treatment response studies is the Neuropsychiatric Inventory (NPI) (Cummings et al. 1994). A validated version is also available for administration by staff for people with dementia who live in nursing homes NPI-NH (Lange et al. 2004).

A major challenge for non-pharmacological intervention studies seeking objective measurement of the enabling interventions included in this chapter is that most interventions have a modest effect and assessing benefits meaningfully is complex and difficult due to the progressive nature of the illness (Katona et al. 2007). Furthermore preoccupation with clinical parameters distracts from capturing the broader impacts on life and living with dementia.

It would seem reasonable to suggest that the influence of an intervention on a person's quality of a person's life is one of the key determinants of an intervention's worth. However, the abstract nature of quality of life (QoL) limits its direct use to people with cognitive capacity so this would tend to exclude people who are no longer able to express themselves verbally. Having examined the associations between commonly used dementia outcome measures and quality of life Banerjee et al (2010) concluded that simple proxy substitution with constructs such as cognitive level or functional ability was inappropriate as such strategies could lead to erroneous conclusions. They recommended use of dementia sensitive QoL measures. Examples of such tools include the 28-item DEMQOL completed by the person with dementia that can be used with people with mild to moderate dementia (MMSE of greater than or equal to 10). The 31-item DEMQOL-Proxy can be completed by carers across the severity spectrum from mild to severe dementia (Smith et al. 2005).

More recent research by Brown (2017) advocates capturing the embodied voice of the person with severe dementia to reflect quality in their life or moment. This, Brown explains, is only possible with a nuanced and shared understanding of the individual's expressive body language and intentional noticing. The importance of knowing both the person and their family and of understanding both the personal and relational dimensions of care and its outcomes is endorsed by Macbride et al. (2017).

Increasingly policy and integrated practice is beginning to embrace personal outcomes (Alzheimer Scotland 2012). This means focussing on what matters to individuals and families and planning how to reach these personal outcomes (Cook and Miller, 2012). The drive towards personal outcomes in dementia care in Scotland is core to the Carers (Scotland) Act 2016 (Scottish Government 2016).

As Miller and Barrie (2016) contend, to do this will require us to move away from a checklist or measurement preoccupation, towards a partnership approach that is conversational. Using techniques such as emotional touch points (Dewar 2010) to enable people to share what is important to them is likely to yield a deeper understanding of the range of influences of enabling interventions within dementia care.

Box 15.2 Reflective questions

- When you review the contribution of a caring intervention for a person with dementia, what evidence do you use to form your view in practice?
- How easy is it to gain the perspective of the person with advanced dementia, and how much do you rely on the views of others?

Reminiscence interventions

Reminiscence is a common approach used within dementia care and it is important to distinguish between the spontaneous forms of reminiscence that occur as a natural part of story-telling and conversations with others (informal) and intentional planned reminiscence activities (formal). Both strategies make important contributions within dementia care as they are affirming strategies that tap into a person's preserved abilities. Reminiscence can be provided on an individual or group basis, be focussed on a particular topic such as a sport e.g. football or baseball (Tolson et al, 2013; Wingbermuehle et al. 2014) or tailored to individual interests (Van Bogaert et al. 2013; 2016).

Evidence of the therapeutic potential of reminiscence is growing and a recent meta-analysis demonstrates that benefits to both cognition and depressive symptoms (Huang et al. 2015). Favourable effects have also been shown on agitation and dysphoria (Low et al. 2015). Other studies highlight a range of observed benefits including positive impacts on verbal communication, expressions of joy and pride, positive anticipation (Coll-Planas et al. 2017). Although it would seem logical to include carers in therapeutic reminiscence a major trial by Woods et al. (2012) that involved 487 caring dyads (person with dementia and family carer) reported an increase in carer stress and anxiety and unexpectedly showed no difference in measured outcomes for individuals between the control and intervention group, although feedback was very positive.

Overall, however, there is growing evidence that reminiscence tailored to an individual's interests can be both enjoyable and helpful. An advantage of group based approaches, particularly where these are planned around shared interests such as football, is the potential to alleviate a sense of loneliness that unfortunately is all too often part of the experience of life with dementia (Coll-Planas et al. 2017).

What is clear from the literature is that reminiscence therapy requires skilful facilitation, planning and management.

Figure 15.2 sets out principles for practice developed from recent football reminiscence studies (Tolson et al. 2013), which can be adapted by practitioners planning reminiscence activities.

Complementary therapies and advanced dementia care

Complementary therapies such as massage, reflexology and aromatherapy (Van Den Bulck and Clusters 2010), offer non-pharmacological alternatives within dementia care. Although there is a paucity of research evidence for their use in advanced dementia a recent mixed method action research study by Mitchell (2018) has demonstrated the practical utility of massage, reflexology, and aromatherapy, within the care of nursing home residents with late stage dementia. Outcomes derived from the Neuropsychiatric Inventory Scale – Nursing Home (Lange et al. 2004) showed a reduction in neuropsychiatric behaviours of nine out of ten residents (Mitchell 2018). The resident who displayed an increased in NPI-NH scores was diagnosed with delirium. Qualitative data from staff and visiting family, demonstrated that the selected complementary therapies showed that such interventions were possible in practice but required input from a qualified Complementary Therapist, and were generally thought to be beneficial for residents. An unexpected finding from this study was the potential of the complimentary therapies to alleviate loneliness was a major determinant of staff selection of residents for participation in the study.

Figure 15.3 offers practice based guidance for the use of individualised complementary therapy within a nursing home environment for residents with advanced dementia drawing on Mitchell's (2018) innovative study.

Principles and practice tips for football focussed reminiscence with people with dementia
The following guidance is aimed at groups or organisations considering establishing a football reminiscence programme for people with dementia. As a starting point it should be recognised that enthusiasm must be coupled with the necessary structures and resources to implement the appropriate supporting policies and procedures referred to in this guide.
Facilitation Reminiscence facilitation may be undertaken by health and social care practitioners and or volunteers with appropriate dementia care skills, training and supervision. The therapeutic intention of the session will determine the required mix of practitioners, volunteers and balance between dementia expertise and understanding of football. Facilitator training should aim to develop: • An understanding of the purpose and benefit of reminiscence activity. • An understanding of dementia and keeping participants safe. • Appreciation of person-centred approaches. • Understanding of the intervention approach and protocol. • Selection and effective use of archive materials. • Ability to plan enjoyable activities appropriate to participants' abilities and interests.
The reminiscence venue • The aesthetics and physical design of the venue should be dementia-friendly. • Football related artefacts should be displayed to provide visual cues. • The venue should be large enough to accommodate between 6 to 12 people including wheelchair users with appropriate furniture to engage in table top activities. • The same venue should available at the same time each week for the duration of the programme (for example at least 12 weeks).
Intervention planning (group based) • Group membership should be consistent and comprise of between 4-12 people with dementia. • The same facilitator and helpers should manage sessions. • An evaluation plan and methods should be agreed and appropriate consents obtained. • 12 week programmes with weekly sessions allow for evaluation of individual benefit • Sessions should be structured with a predictable format of activities to open and close the session. • Activities should be varied at a pace appropriate to members of the group and might include-songs, photographic and visual image elicited reminiscence, artefact tactile or sensory stimulation of memories such as through smells and sounds.
Monitoring and evaluation Individual experience is central to evaluation; feedback from the person with dementia and their carer and staff is important. The behaviour and mood of the person with dementia, vocalisation, facial expression, engagement and body language are all indicative of a persontțs response and interest in the reminiscence activities.

Figure 15.2 Football focussed reminiscence principles and practice tips

Conclusion

As there is currently no cure or effective treatment for dementia it is important that we develop approaches and interventions that help to preserve a person's abilities, reduce distress and promote a sense of well-being. There is much we have to learn in terms of both therapeutic outcomes and personal outcomes to guide us in the delivery and evaluation of the usefulness of caring interventions with

Preparation for complementary therapy

It is first important to:

Establish if the nursing home is able to accommodate complementary therapy. Questions to ask yourself are;:

Does the nursing home have a quiet space where the intervention can take place?
Is this space:

    Free from distraction?
    Free from noise?
    Well lit?
    A safe and secure environment for the resident?

Note tthsome complementary therapy interventions can be provided in a group setting but the provider/therapist must ensure that the resident's dignity and privacy are respected.

Establish if complementary therapy is the right intervention for the resident.
Questions to ask yourself are:

How does the resident feel about complementary therapy?
    Are they accepting of, unsure, or against the idea?

Note – for a person that is unable to verbalise their thoughts, use visual and tactile techniques (demonstrative ideas, pictures).

Are there any preferences that the resident may have?
    Do they like a particular type of intervention?
    Do they enjoy touch/contact?
    Do they have a preference of smell, cream, or oil?

Note – use a collaborative approach. Communicate with the resident, their family and friends, and use their individual profiles to help select a complementary therapy

Delivering Complementary Therapy

Remember to:

Make a connection with the resident
Always try to connect with the resident. Be it connecting with, eye contact, verbally, or tactfully. Find something you have in common or something that will ground the complementary therapy session.

Engage throughout the session
Try to make the resident feel as comfortable as possible by engaging with them. Offer reassurance, and gain reassurance. Make sure they know what is happening and what you are doing.

Build a relationship/rapport
This is a prime opportunity to really get to know the resident. It is one to one time with you and them – Make it count.

Manual pressure
Be mindful of the pressure you use on the resident's skin. Older skin is thinner and can tear easily (Holmes et al. 2013), so you must ensure that the pressure you apply is appropriate to the residents and that the skin is

moisturised enough. The movement should glide and be soft. If the skin drags or sticks, there isn't enough cream or oil being used.

Concluding the complementary therapy session

Finish by:

Ending on a good note
Don't end the session abruptly. Try to ensure the resident is aware that the session has ended. Reflect with the resident on how they felt the session was. Did the enjoy it? What did they like? How do they feel now?

Reflecting on the session.
By reflecting on the session with the resident, you can learn and build on the therapeutic experience. This will make the session more enjoyable, and truly memorable for the resident.

Figure 15.3 Delivering complementary therapy within nursing homes

individuals. What is clear from the reviewed evidence is that caring interventions have much to offer people with dementia and while researchers deliberate verifiable outcomes, in practice and family caring the benefits to individuals in the moment of care are often apparent to those who listen to the person or can interpret their embodied expression.

References

Alzheimer's Scotland (2012) "Delivering Integrated Dementia Care: the 8 Pillars Model of Community Support." Available from: http://www.alzscot.org/assets/0000/4613/FULL_REPORT_8_Pillars_Model_of_Community_Support.pdf.

Brown, M. (2017) "Multiple perspectives on the quality of life of people with severe dementia living in a care home: A collective case study approach." University of the West of Scotland: Unpublished PhD Thesis.

Coll-Planas, L., Watchman, K., Doménech, S., McGillivray, D., O'Donnell, H. and Tolson, D. (2017) "Developing evidence for football (soccer) reminiscence interventions with long-term care: a cooperative approach applied in Scotland and Spain." *Journal of the American Medical Directors Association*, 18(4): 355–360. doi:10.1016/j.jamda.2017.01.013.

Cook, A. and Miller, E. (2012) "Talking Points. Personal Outcomes Approach." Available from: http://www.jitscotland.org.uk/wp-content/uploads/2014/01/Talking-Points-Practical-Guide-21-June-2012.pdf.

Cui, Y., Shen, M., Ma, Y. and Wen, S.W., (2017) "Senses make sense: An individualized multisensory stimulation for dementia." *Medical Hypotheses*, 98:11–14.

Cummings, J.L., Mega, M., Gray, K., Rosenberg-Thompson, S., Carusi, D.A. and Gornbein, J. (1994) "The Neuropsychiatric Inventory: comprehensive assessment of psychopathology in dementia." *Neurology*, 44: 2308–2314.

Dewar, B., Mackay, R., Smith, S., Pullin, S. and Tocher, R. (2010) "Use of emotional touchpoints as a method of tapping into the experience of receiving compassionate care in a hospital setting." *Journal of Nursing Research*, 15: 29–41.

Holmes, R.F., Davidson, M.W., Thompson, B.J. and Kelechi, T.J. (2013) "Skin tears: care and management of the older adult at home." *Home Healthcare Now*, 31(2): 90–101.

Huang, H.C., Chen, Y.T. andChen, P.Y. (2015) "Reminiscence therapy improves cognitive functions and reduces depressive symptoms in elderly people with dementia: A meta-analysis of randomized controlled trials." *Journal of the American Medical Directors Association*, 16: 1087–1094.

Katona, C., Livingston, G., Cooper, C., Ames, D., Brodaty, H. and Chiu, E. (on behalf of the Consensus Group). (2007) "International Psychogeriatric Association consensus statement on defining and measuring treatment benefits in dementia." *International Psychogeriatrics*, 19(3): 345–354.

Lange, R.T., Hopp, G.A. andKang, N., (2004) "Psychometric properties and factor structure of the neuropsychiatric inventory nursing home version in an elderly neuropsychiatric population." *International Journal of Geriatric Psychiatry*, 19: 440–448.

Low, L.F., Baker, J.R. and Harrison, F. (2015) "The Lifestyle Engagement Activity Program (LEAP): Implementing social and recreational activity into case-managed homecare." *Journal of American Medical Directors Association*, 16: 1069–1076.

Macbride, T., Miller, E. and Dewar, B. (2017) "'I know who I am; the real me, and that will come back.' The importance of relational practice in improving outcomes for carers of people with dementia." *Illness, Crisis and Loss*. Available from: http://journals.sagepub.com/doi/full/10.1177/1054137317700061.

Miller, E. and Barrie, K. (2016) *Learning from the Meaningful and Measurable project: strengthening links between identity, action and decision-making*. Glasgow: Health Improvement Scotland. Available from: http://ihub.scot/media/1137/20160908-po-learning-key-messages-1-0.pdf.

Mitchell, B. (2018) "The contribution of complementary therapy within the care of nursing home residents experiencing later stage dementia: an action research study. " University of the West of Scotland. Unpublished PhD Thesis.

Scottish Government. (2016) "Carers' Scotland Act." Edinburgh: The Scottish Government.

Smith, S.C., Lamping, D.L., Banerjee, S., Harwood, R., Foley, B., Smith, P., Cook, J.C., Murray, J., Prince, M., Levin, E., Mann, A. and Knapp, M. (2005) "Measurement of health related quality of life for people with dementia: development of a new instrument (DEMQOL) and an evaluation of current methodology." *Health Technology Assessment*, 9(10): 1–108.

Spector, A. and Orrell, M. (2010) "Using a bio-psychosocial model of dementia as a tool to guide clinical practice." *International Psychogeriatrics*, 22(6): 957–965.

Tolson, D., Lowndes, A. and O'Donnell, H. (2013) "Harnessing the heritage of football; Creating meaningful activities and therapeutic reminiscence work with people with dementia." Available from: http://www.ahrc.ac.uk/research/readwatchlisten/filmsandpodcasts/memoriesfchertiageoffootball.

Van Bogaert, P., Van Grinsven, R. and Tolson, D. (2013) "A feasibility trial of individual reminiscence based on the SolCos Model for people with mild to moderate dementia." *Journal of American Directors Association*, 14(7): 528–529.

Van Bogaert, P., Tolson, D. and Eerlingen, R. (2016) "SolCos model-based individual reminiscence for older adults with mild to moderate dementia in nursing homes: A randomized controlled intervention study." *Journal of Psychiatry Mental Health Nursing*, 23: 568–575.

Van den Bulck, J. and Custers, K. (2010) "Belief in complementary and alternative medicine is related to age and paranormal beliefs in adults." *The European Journal of Public Health*, 20 (2): 227–230.

Wingbermuehle, C., Bryer, D. and Berg-Weger, M. (2014) "Baseball reminiscence league: A model for supporting persons with dementia." *Journal of American Medical Directors Association*, 15: 85–89.

Further reading

Care Inspectorate. (2016) "Promoting positive outcomes for people living with dementia." Available from: http://hub.careinspectorate.com/media/310905/promoting-outcomes-for-people-living-with-dementia-2-.pdf.

Lee, H. and Adams, T. (eds) (2011) *Creative approaches in dementia care.* Hampshire: Palgrave Macmillan.

My Home Life CYMRU. (2014) "Getting to know you: A guide for reminiscence and life story work with older people living in care homes. " Available from: http://myhomelife.org.uk/wp-content/uploads/2014/11/MHL-CYMRU-GETTING-TO-KNOW-YOU.pdf.

Tay, S. (2014) *Complementary Therapies for Older People in Care.* London and Philadelphia: Singing Dragon.

16 Psychiatric symptoms in dementia

Paul Brown, Adam Daly and Graham A. Jackson

Introduction

Dementia is not a disease in itself, rather it is a syndrome with a collection of signs and symptoms that can be caused by many different disease processes. People will often think of dementia as causing problems with the way the brain works, for example in memory, language, making sense of the world around you and being able to do every day tasks. It is well established that as the disease progresses these type of symptoms also get worse.

However there are another group of symptoms that can sometimes be even more disruptive to a person and cause even more distress. These symptoms and signs, as a group, are given many different names and are listed in Table 16.1 below:

As with many mental health disorders the symptoms are influenced by changes in environmental factors, medical conditions, psychological approaches and by social situations. Considering dementia broadly in this way is called a "biopsychosocial" way of thinking. There are similarities with other mental health disorders that we can use in both identification of symptoms and to guide treatment and monitor response to treatment. However, given the wide variety of factors that influence the symptoms, each person presents with unique problems and therefore this requires a person-centred approach.

Some confusion can arise within clinical teams when thinking about the terminology for these conditions. Historically terms that have been used have included "challenging behaviour" and "behaviour that challenges", and the medical literature has used and continues to use "behavioural and psychological symptoms of dementia" (BPSD). A current popular term is "stress and distress", indicating that the psychiatric symptoms have a stressful impact on those caring for the person with dementia, and supporting the person who is caring is every bit as important as supporting a person with dementia. Each of these terms has their pros and cons and they remain useful in communicating and describing clinical features when working within multidisciplinary teams. There is a danger in clinical practice that using these terms too freely when considering an individual means that we miss the unique points in that person's care and fail to be person-centred. For clarity and consistency in this chapter however, the term BPSD will be used when discussing these symptoms as a group.

Box 16.1 Reflective thought

Think about how some of the symptoms of dementia, particularly those referred to as psychiatric or psychological symptoms, are referred to. Even within this book, different terms are used, largely dependent on the professional group of the chapter authors. Terms include stress and distress associated with dementia, behavioural and psychological symptoms of dementia and challenging behaviour. Think about how such labelling may influence how these actions are dealt with, particularly in terms of tolerance and acceptance, and the use of social, environmental, pharmaceutical and non-pharmaceutical approaches.

Regardless of what terminology is used, and whether we consider each symptom individually or as a group, it is vital that the person with dementia is not being labelled as "badly behaved" or "attention seeking". Although occasionally still mentioned in some settings, these views are unhelpful in trying to understand and help. More appropriate explanations include that the person with dementia is attempting to communicate their distress to the people around them or that they are experiencing psychotic, mood or other symptoms as a result of changes within their brain.

BPSD symptoms are not unusual; they are very common and indeed to some extent the symptoms may be seen as a normal part of dementia, occurring at some point in 80 to 90% of people with dementia (Nowrangi et al. 2015). At any point, 61% of people with dementia who live in the community have such symptoms (Lyketsos et al. 2000) and in care homes this rises to 79% (Margallo-Lana et al. 2001). This is particularly relevant when we are considering institutional care, as it tends to be this rather than a decline in functioning which leads to admission (Wancata et al. 2003), largely due to the impact on levels of caregiver stress (Tan et al. 2005). BPSD can also indicate a worsening of underlying dementia and can give a prognosis towards more rapid progression (Paulsen et al. 2000).

The fact that BPSD is common, distressing and difficult to treat has contributed to an increase in the profile of the specialty of old-age psychiatry in the United Kingdom. Psychiatrists work alongside a wide range of other professionals including nurses, allied health professions, social workers and other medical colleagues. Psychiatrists routinely see people who have problems with for example, mood, hallucinations, delusions, anxiety and sleep problems. These problems can be found in a variety of conditions, including dementia. The consultant old age psychiatrist

Table 16.1 Psychiatric features of dementia

Learning point: Some psychiatric features of dementia

Agitation

Low mood (or dysphoria)

Aggression

Apathy

Irritability or lability of affect

Psychosis (principally hallucinations and delusions)

Sleep disturbance

Wandering

Hoarding

Disinhibition – socially and sexually inappropriate behaviour

provides clinical leadership to the multidisciplinary team. The core remit of the multidisciplinary team is the assessment and accurate diagnosis of dementia (and other mental health conditions in older adults) and effective management of these conditions.

When a health professional begins to assess the patient who has BPSD they must be aware of the complex interactions between the dementia, acute medical issues, psychological factors, social factors and environmental issues.

Assessment of the causes of BPSD

The role of underlying dementia

The various and wide ranging functions of the brain can be dependent on several different areas, and as a dementia progresses symptoms can present in a variety of ways because of this. For example, if the frontal lobes of the brain are involved this can cause problems with organisational, planning and decision-making skills as well as affecting judgement and personality. Widespread vascular disease is often linked to depression (Baldwin & O'Brien 2002). It is helpful to consider in addition to changes in the structure of the larger part of the brain there are also changes in the chemical transmitters between nerve cells (neurotransmitters). Serotonin and noradrenaline (Lai et al. 2011; Weinshenker 2008) for example, are chemicals that we know are important in the regulation of mood (many antidepressants target these chemicals too) and so we can begin to understand why changes in mood happen in dementia. Alterations in the neurotransmitters dopamine and acetylcholine can be related to apathy (David et al. 2008). Reductions in dopamine are also seen in dementia with Lewy Bodies along with a range of other chemical and structural changes that could be responsible for visual hallucinations being more common in this condition than other forms of dementia (Taylor et al. 2011).

The role of precipitating factors

In this section factors that may precipitate and perpetuate BPSD in people with dementia will be outlined. Such factors can be categorised into biological, psychological and social/environmental factors.

Biological factors

A person with dementia can experience a worsening of their mental health with relatively minor physical health issues. As these often do not cause problems in people without dementia, they can be overlooked when they occur in people with dementia. Common examples seen in practice include untreated or undertreated pain, infection, errors with medication or excessive medication/intolerance, constipation, hunger, thirst or tiredness. These factors may also lead to delirium; the presence of dementia is a high risk factor for delirium (this is discussed further in Chapter 18).

Any person assessing BPSD must carry out a comprehensive clinical assessment to identify any medical factors that can be treated, often resulting in significant improvement in the mental health of the person as a consequence.

Psychological factors

A number of psychological theories have been proposed regarding BPSD. Although as previously stated, the causes are likely to be complex and in many situations there are multiple causes, it can be useful to think in terms of some symptoms of BPSD as an attempt to communicate an unmet need. Thinking about this, basic needs must be met before more complex ones are possible. In this theory physical health needs have to be met first before we can move on to others. After this, one can consider needs for feelings of safety and security. If these are met one can consider the need for relationships, friends and a sense of belonging. This way of thinking is based on Maslow's hierarchy of needs (Maslow 1943) with physiological needs at the bottom of the hierarchy with the type of need increasing in complexity until self-actualisation is sought and attained at the top.

Box 16.2 Practice point

There are often unmet needs in dementia care. Common unmet needs are thirst, hunger, untreated pain, constipation, loneliness, abandonment and isolation, as well as lack of stimulation, or distress from overstimulation.

These particular needs have been chosen as examples because at a practical level, they can often be addressed with resultant improvement in the level of distress in the person. As part of a holistic assessment, one must try to determine what the unmet needs are of a person in distress and work creatively with the team to deliver personalised care to meet the specific need(s).

Environmental and social factors

These factors affect one's ability to make sense of the surrounding space. There are numerous changes that can be made to improve the environment of a person with dementia – many may not be immediately obvious. For example as we age we need more light in order to see clearly, and so a dimly lit room may not be cosy to a person with dementia but rather it could appear very dark and frightening. Floors that are indistinct from walls (the same colour for example), could give the appearance of a floor that goes on forever. Important social aspects include the quality and appropriateness of inter-personal relationships and the level of occupation and stimulation given to the person within the care environment.

Box 16.3 Practice point: Common environmental issues

- Poor lighting
- High levels of often unrecognisable noise
- Too hot or too cold
- Lack of wall/floor distinction
- Highly patterned floors
- Poor signage

Specific symptoms

When assessing BPSD, specific symptoms should be looked for. These symptoms can be identified and communicated to others, and form therapeutic targets when treatment is undertaken. The descriptive terms listed below can be supplemented and improved by using objective measures such as the Challenging Behaviour Scale (CBS).

- Agitation: Agitation is classically the physical sign of anxiety (for example, worry and apprehension), however in dementia it is often expanded to include other features and indeed can become synonymous with the term BPSD. If we are to think about agitation as a separate symptom, the person often experiences an inability to sit still. They frequently shake and move their limbs. Agitation may also take the form of shouting or screaming. Agitation may respond only briefly from reassurance or not at all.

- Aggression: Aggression varies widely in how it presents, from harsh words to serious physical assaults. It is regularly brought to the attention of services when carers and family members feel risk has increased. There has often been a degree of verbal and/or physical aggression taking place for some time prior to the presentation frequently this behaviour is not in keeping with a person's previous history or personality. Aggression is perhaps the symptom in dementia with the highest risk and it is the only BPSD symptom for which antipsychotic medication is licensed.

- Depression, low mood or dysphoria: Depressive disorder often precedes a developing dementia. A person with depression may be misdiagnosed as having a dementia. Changes in mood (including lowering of mood) are common in dementia and the symptoms can often be difficult to tell apart, especially in the early stages of the illness. When assessing a person with ongoing low mood, it can be useful to gauge other symptoms that one would connect to a depressive illness (a diurnal variation, poor appetite, early morning wakening and low motivation for example). It is extremely important to accurately detect a depressive illness (which can also cause memory and other cognitive problems) because effective treatment may bring about substantial improvement in the person. Depression itself can lead to significant challenges for a person with dementia and their care network including reduced oral intake and activity. Depression that causes significant cognitive impairment and a dementia-like picture in an older adult is sometimes referred to as depressive pseudo-dementia.

- Apathy: As opposed to depression, where one has a low mood, apathy instead indicates ambivalence and a reduction in emotional responses overall. This has been described in several different types of dementia, making apathy is a very common finding, and is hard to treat effectively.

- Irritability or liability of affect: These features can be linked to aggression or low mood, but the risk can sometimes be reduced by acknowledging and planning for how to manage episodes when problems occur.

- Psychosis: Psychosis encompasses a wide range of abnormal beliefs and perceptions. These include delusions (a fixed, usually false belief that persists in a person even when there is clear evidence to the contrary – which include misidentification) and hallucinations (a perception without a stimulus). It is important to acknowledge the difference in these terms as they have different causes and different treatments. Hallucinations are common in all dementias in the later stages how-ever, it is important to note that in Lewy body dementia visual hallucinations are often prominent in the early stages. This is highly relevant because medication one might normally propose in such a situation (antipsychotics) carry a much greater risk of serious side effects in people with Lewy body dementia. Therefore, efforts are made to avoid antipsychotics completely in this patient group and indeed their symptoms may well respond effectively to other classes of medication. If anti-psychotics are deemed essential, only certain drugs are specially selected and they are used with caution.

Box 16.4 Learning point: Examples of misidentification issues

- Capgras syndrome: a known person is replaced by an imposter
- Fregoli syndrome: strangers appear as if a known person
- Agnosia: the inability to recognise people or objects

- Sleep disturbance: A more frequent feature as the condition progresses, the gradual loss of some aspects of the circadian rhythm is well recognised – in extreme examples leading to a person with dementia being awake sometimes for days at a time. This can be especially distressing to carers as it can lead to a loss of sleep for all involved.
- Wandering: An often misused term, wandering implies active movement (usually walking) without a goal or aim. In cases where there is a goal or aim, then this is not wandering and can often be more easily understood. As with other symptoms, it is useful to be clear about the precise nature of the symp-tom so that it might guide management. The wandering can have many driving factors, such as a desire to exercise, to explore or as a manifestation of agita-tion with an inability to remain still.
- Disinhibition: This symptom can also vary widely, ranging from out of character comments about a person's attire or build to potentially dangerous sexual disin-hibition. People with fronto-temporal dementia are particularly affected by these types of symptoms. In such situations the risk to others (and to the person with dementia) must be taken into account when determining the speed and content of a treatment package.

Management

The management of BPSD should always begin with a detailed assessment of symp-toms whilst identifying any precipitating or perpetuating factors that could be remedied.

It is very important to obtain a full account from the relative/main carer about the symptoms the person with dementia has, and how it impacts on them. The relative/carer spends considerable periods of time with the person who has dementia and hence their descriptions of current and past problems can be incredibly valuable.

The severity of the symptoms, the stress the person and their carers experience and the risk posed to all involved will guide the speed and composition of the treatment plan being implemented.

General principles in managing BPSD are that a person-centred approach must be used, and non-pharmacological approaches should be used first as these are less likely to cause harm then pharmacological approaches in general. Medication is generally reserved for people with dementia who do not respond to non-drug based approaches. However, there are some important clinical situations whereby medication has an important role. These include patients with prominent, distressing psychotic symptoms or significant depression. In addition, medication is used in other situations when the person is very distressed and not responding to other approaches. Medication can also be very important in scenarios whereby there is significant risk to the person or others.

Non-pharmacological treatment

Although such methods should be considered as first-line the evidence for these is sadly lacking. At present, the strongest evidence is for supporting family and caregivers, primarily aimed at education and increasing resilience in this group. This reflects the importance of family and caregivers in the management and support of a person with dementia. Interventions with a limited evidence base include aromatherapy, reminiscence, therapy, validation, light therapy and acupuncture. It is worth noting that none of these is likely to cause substantial harm and that what works for one individual may not necessarily work for another so it is important to keep care plans person-centred.

For more complex situations, formal psychological techniques based around a person-centred approach have also been shown to be of benefit. The Newcastle Model (James 2011) relies on the theory of unmet needs and has been implemented in settings including specialist community teams and inpatient psychiatry wards. Such techniques require specific training and ongoing support to ensure that not just the principles of the psychological intervention are adhered to but also that the model itself is implemented consistently.

Pharmacological treatment

Historically medication has been used often and liberally to manage the behavioural and psychological symptoms of dementia. However, there is now evidence that several of these medications, most notably antipsychotics, have a significant potential for harm. Efforts are currently underway to reduce the amount of psychotropics (medications that alter mental function) prescribed to people with dementia, but it must be stressed that these medications still do have an important role to play in appropriate patients and clinical situations. This is discussed further in Chapter 18.

Conclusion

Behavioural and psychological symptoms of dementia are common, complex and challenging. They are a very important cause of carer stress and admission into institutional care and deserve higher levels of research attention.

Professionals helping patients and their families with these symptoms must adopt a person-centred, fully holistic approach to assessment and treatment thereby optimising outcomes.

References

Baldwin, R.C. and O'Brien, J. (2002) "Vascular basis of late-onset depressive disorder. British Journal of Psychiatry." *Psychopharmacology*, 180: 157–160.

David, R.I., Koulibaly, M., Benoit, M., Garcia, R., Caci, H., Darcourt, J. and Robert, P. (2008) "Striatal dopamine transporter levels correlate with apathy in neurodegenerative diseases A SPECT study with partial volume effect correction." *Clinical Neurology and Neurosurgery*, 110(1): 19–24.

James, I. (2011) *Understanding Behaviour in Dementia That Challenges: A Guide to Assessment and Treatment.* London: Jessica Kingsley.

Konovalov, S.I., Muralee, S. and Tampi, R.R. (2008) "Anticonvulsants for the treatment of behavioral and psychological symptoms of dementia: a literature review." *International Psychogeriatrics*, 20(2): 293–308.

Lai, M.K.P., Tsang, S.W., Esiri, M.M., Francis, P.T., Wong, P.T.H. and Chen, C.P. (2011) "Differential involvement of hippocampal serotonin1A receptors and re-uptake sites in non-cognitive behaviors of Alzheimer's disease." *Psychopharmacology*, 213: 431–443.

Lyketsos, CG, Steinberg, M., Tschanz, J.T., Norton, M.C., Steffens, D.C. and Breitner, J.C. (2000) "Mental and behavioral disturbances in dementia: findings from Cache County Study on Memory and Aging." *American Journal of Psychiatry*, 157: 708–714.

Margallo-Lana, M.I., Swann, A., O'Brien, J., Fairbairn, A., Reichelt, K., Potkins, D., Mynt, P. and Ballard, C. (2001) "Prevalence and pharmacological management of behavioural and psychological symptoms amongst dementia sufferers living in care environments." *International Journal of Geriatric Psychiatry*, 16(1): 39–44.

Maslow, A.H. (1943) "A theory of human motivation." *Psychological Review*, 50(4): 370–396.

Norwangi, M.A., Lyketsos, C. and Rosenberg, P.B. (2015) "Principles and management of neuropsychiatric symptoms in Alzheimer's dementia." *Alzheimer's research and therapy*, 7: 12.

Paulsen, J.S.L., Salmon, D.P., Thal, L.J., Romero, R., Weisstein-Jenkins, C., Galasko, D., Hofstetter, C.R., Thomas, R., Grant, I. and Jeste, D.V. (2000) "Incidence of and risk factors for hallucinations and delusions in patients with probable AD." *Neurology*, 54(10): 1965–1971.

Tan, L.L., Wong, H.B. and Allen, H. (2005) "The impact of neuropsychiatric symptoms of dementia on distress in family and professional caregivers in Singapore." *International Psychogeriatrics*, 17(2): 253–263.

Taylor, J.P., Firbank, M., Barnett, N., Pearce, P., Livingstone, A., Mosimann, U., Eyre. J., McKeith, I.G. and O'Brien, J.T. (2011) "Visual hallucinations in dementia with Lewy bodies: transcranial magnetic stimulation study." *British Journal of Psychiatry*, 199(6): 492–500. doi:10.1192/bjp.bp.110.090373.

Wancata, J., Windhaber, J., Krautgartner, M. and Alexandrowicz, R. (2003) "The consequences of non-cognitive symptoms of dementia in medical hospital departments." *The International Journal of Psychiatry in Medicine*, 33(3): 257–271.

Weinshenker, D.I. (2008) "Functional consequences of locus coeruleus degeneration in Alzheimer's disease." *Current Alzheimer Research*, 5(3): 342–345.

Further reading

Banerjee, S. (2009) "Report on the prescribing of anti-psychotic drugs to people with dementia." Department of Health, UK Government. Available from: http://webarchive.nationalarchives. gov.uk/20130107105354/http:/www.dh.gov.uk/en/Publicationsandstatistics/Publications/Publica tionsPolicyAndGuidance/DH_108303.

Greener, M. (2017) "New insights into delusional misidentification syndromes." *Progress in Neurology and Psychiatry*, 21(2): 33–35.

James, I. (2011) *Understanding Behaviour in Dementia That Challenges: A Guide to Assessment and Treatment.* London: Jessica Kingsley.

17 Medication and dementia

Guy Holloway and Lucy Stirland

Introduction

A number of particular issues arise in the use of medication in people with dementia. There are several drugs licensed for dementia but they are of only modest benefit in most patients. Despite considerable research regrettably there are, as yet, no agents available which have been shown to reliably inhibit the progression of most dementia pathologies. The focus of drug treatment thus remains on treating the symptoms, whether these be cognitive, behavioural or psychiatric, and by default is therefore essentially palliative.

Since the 1990s there has been increasing concern that certain medications, particularly antipsychotics and drugs with anticholinergic activity, can have adverse effects on people with dementia (Richardson et al. 2018). More recently the issue of medication reducing the risk of dementia has received more attention; rightly so since some estimates suggest that delaying the average age of onset of dementia by five years might reduce the number of people with the condition by one third (Alzheimer's Research UK 2015).

The decision whether or not to prescribe a drug for someone with any condition appears at first straightforward. The doctor diagnoses the condition, there is a drug available for the condition, the doctor prescribes the drug that the patient then takes reliably and the patient therefore benefits. However prescribing decisions are rarely this simple, and perhaps nowhere less so than for people with dementia. Every decision to prescribe requires a careful risk-benefit analysis, weighing up the potential benefits of the drug to that individual against the potential adverse effects, and then communicating that to the patient, their carers or those with legal authority to make decisions on their behalf, and taking their views into account. This issue is particularly germane when considering the use of restrictive measures to enforce treatment, such as covert administration or use of mental health or capacity legislation.

Modern medicine continually aspires to refine practice to become more evidence-based. Regrettably much of the so-called evidence base is contaminated by flawed and biased studies, many of which are now easily available to patients on the internet. Uncritical and untrained evaluation of the evidence can lead to poor decision-making and adverse outcomes for patients. This is particularly the case for studies of drug interventions, the majority of which are still funded by drug companies who have a vested interest in demonstrating the efficacy of their products in order to sell more. Studies of non-pharmacological alternatives usually have to compete for funding from overstretched non-commercial research budgets.

Publication bias results from studies that show positive outcomes being more likely to be published than those showing null or negative outcomes (Guyatt et al. 2011). Various initiatives have sought to counter this. Cochrane[1] is an independent, non-profit, non-governmental organisation which seeks to promote evidence-based medicine through conducting systematic reviews of randomised controlled trials. AllTrials[2] is an organisation which campaigns for the registration of all medical studies and open access to data.

The older we get, the less able we are to clear drugs from our bodies. Figure 17.2 shows decreasing rates of creatinine clearance by the kidneys with increasing age. Creatinine is a waste product of metabolism that the kidneys filter out of blood. Creatinine clearance is therefore a measure of the kidneys' ability to filter blood. The kidneys are an important route of elimination of drugs from the body and similar variations with increasing age will occur with other routes.

People with dementia often have comorbid physical conditions affecting their sensitivity to medication, are more likely to be on multiple medications with thus an increased risk of drug interactions and have a condition which will lead to increasing sensitivity of their brains to the adverse effects of medications over time.

Well-considered analysis of the risks of treatment weighed against the potential benefit is at the core of ethical and safe prescribing. Such a risk-benefit analysis must be person-centred and take account of all the factors illustrated in Figure 17.1. People with dementia do by definition have a condition that is almost certainly going to deteriorate over time. Their situation is thus dynamic and changing so a medication which may be necessary and appropriate at one point in their illness course may not be so at another point. Distressing symptoms such as agitation, anxiety or depression may come and go independent of drug treatment, and often are more dependent on environmental and psychological factors. Care must be taken not to erroneously attribute resolution of such symptoms to coincidental drug prescription; neither should patients be denied a treatment which has been of clear overall benefit to them.

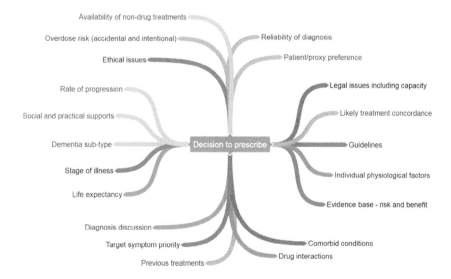

Figure 17.1 Factors influencing the decision to prescribe and the timing of prescription

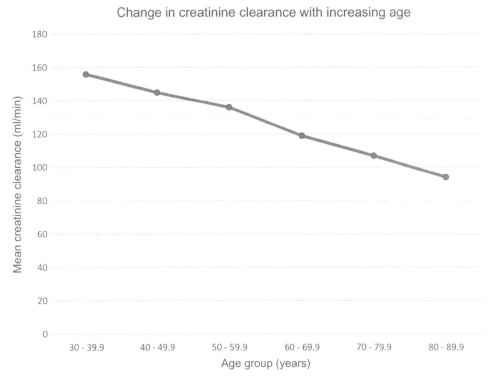

Figure 17.2 Change in creatinine clearance with increasing age
Source: Adapted from (Glassock and Winearls 2009).

Historically less attention has been paid to the importance of decisions about when to stop prescribing medications, although increasingly professional guidance is encompassing these issues, especially in palliative care scenarios (O'Mahony et al. 2014).

Dementia prevention

Are there any medications which can prevent people developing dementia in the first place? For some years it was thought that the cholesterol-lowering statin drugs, such as simvastatin and atorvastatin, may reduce the risk of developing dementia. A number of trials have now shown conclusively that they do not (McGuinness et al. 2016). Some drugs used to treat high blood pressure may reduce the risk of developing dementia, although further trials are required to confirm this (Rouch et al. 2015).

It has been known for some time that anti-cholinergic drugs can cause delirium and cognitive impairment in vulnerable individuals. Recent research shows a correlation between duration and extent of exposure to drugs with anti-cholinergic properties, and subsequent risk of developing dementia (Gray et al. 2015). There is also evidence that the strength of anti-cholinergic effect is related to the risk of dementia (Richardson et al. 2018). What we do not know is if stopping these drugs reduces risk, although common sense suggests anti-cholinergic burden should be reduced as much as possible.

Drug treatment of behavioural and psychological symptoms in dementia

Behavioural and psychological symptoms in dementia (BPSD) are common, distressing for the patient and their carers, associated with institutionalisation and can be difficult to treat. For many years antipsychotic drugs have been used to treat behavioural problems in people with dementia.

BPSD can be grouped into four broadly overlapping categories: mood disturbance, agitation, impulse control problems and psychosis. The management of behaviours in each category will usually require different management strategies. One of the potential difficulties with applying trial evidence to clinical practice is that studies by necessity typically use scores on rating scales as outcome measures. Since such scales usually combine multiple different areas of BPSD, a change in the score may represent a marked change in a limited number of behaviours or a modest change in multiple behaviours. Adopting a prioritised problem list can help keep the treatment patient-centred.

Both typical (first generation) and atypical (second generation) antipsychotic drugs do have beneficial effects on agitation in Alzheimer's dementia. However, only about 20% of people treated with antipsychotics will gain benefit from the treatment over and above the effects of placebo (Banerjee 2009).

Box 17.1 Examples of good practice

- Consider alternatives including analgesia and non-drug treatments
- Start with low doses of medication and increase slowly
- Review prescription regularly
- Consider discontinuing antipsychotics after 12 weeks

(Corbett et al. 2014; van der Spek et al. 2018)

The only drug that is currently licensed in the UK for treatment of agitation and aggression in dementia is risperidone. Research has shown that both risperidone and olanzapine are associated with an increased risk of strokes or similar events in people with dementia. The absolute risk remains low, going from roughly 1 in 100 people with dementia experiencing a stroke, or similar event, per year to three in 100. However use of antipsychotics is also associated with many other adverse effects including Parkinson's-like symptoms, walking problems and drops in blood pressure (Corbett et al. 2014). Delirium often complicates, and can worsen, the trajectory of decline in dementia. Antipsychotics, particularly low dose haloperidol and olanzapine, do have a clear role in the management of delirium but care should be taken that when appropriately commenced in hospital they are not inappropriately continued on discharge (Young et al. 2010).

Box 17.2 Reflective point

Voice of Mrs. H., the wife of a gentleman with severe dementia and high-risk distressed behaviour:

> I have had a lot of concerns about the use of antipsychotics, having read about them. I know he has been more settled but I have been concerned when he's been sedated or "absent".

> I have often wondered about a drug holiday but this does scare me because I know how bad things were.
>
> I would like his behaviour controlled without resort to medication. However I accept that if he's really distressed he does need them. I worry his current medication will stop working and he will need more and this will become a pattern.

Given the concerns about the safety of antipsychotics, prescribers will often consider alternatives. Donepezil does not help agitation in Alzheimer's dementia (Howard et al. 2007) but may help anxiety, apathy and depression Feldman et al. 2005). Galantamine may postpone the emergence of BPSD (Tariot et al. 2000). Rivastigmine reduces the likelihood of being prescribed an antipsychotic (Suh et al. 2004). Memantine does not help established agitation but may help other BPSD. A Cochrane review of nine randomised controlled trials (RCTs) suggests modest benefit from serotonin specific reuptake inhibitor (SSRI) antidepressants but also that they have significant side effects, especially increased risk of falls (Seitz et al. 2011). The anti-epileptic and mood-stabilising drugs Carbamazepine and Valproate have been used for agitation. Valproate is of no benefit and appears to accelerate cognitive decline and brain atrophy (Lonergan and Luxenberg 2009; Fleisher et al. 2011). RCTs of Carbamazepine have shown either modest or no benefit and substantial risk of significant side effects (Konovalov et al. 2008). The response of depression in Alzheimer's disease to treatment with antidepressants is poor (Banerjee et al. 2011) but they may reduce longer-term mortality when given in the prodromal stages of the disease (Enache et al. 2016). By contrast, there is some evidence that Trazodone and SSRIs may be of benefit for BPSD in behavioural variant Frontotemporal Dementia (Lebert et al. 2004).

Pain is under-recognised and under-treated in people with dementia although use of rating scales can help improve pain identification. Careful escalation of analgesia in patients unselected for pain yielded similar magnitude of benefit on agitation to antipsychotics (Corbett et al. 2012).

Box 17.3 Tips for good practice

- Offer written information about the medications suggested and allow the patient to make an informed decision in collaboration with their carers and healthcare professionals
- Review patients taking anti-dementia drugs regularly during the initial phases of treatment. The drugs should only be continued if they have an overall worthwhile effect on cognitive, global, functional or behavioural symptoms.
- Consider requesting a medication review when patients are prescribed numerous medications
- Ensure good communication when the patient's care setting changes, for example referring to local medicines reconciliation guidelines (NICE 2015)
- Optimise concordance with treatment by use of aids such as blister packs or medication prompts etc.

Cholinesterase inhibitors and memantine

There are currently four medications licensed in the UK for the treatment of Alzheimer's type dementia. Guidance states that these should only be initiated by a specialist experienced in the management of dementia and this now includes suitably trained GPs, Advanced Nurse Practitioners and nurse prescribers (BNF 2016).

The anti-dementia drugs are acetylcholinesterase inhibitors (donepezil, galantamine and rivastigmine, also called anti-cholinesterases) and an NMDA receptor modulator, memantine.

Levels of acetylcholine are reduced in the brains of people with Alzheimer's disease, and this has been closely linked to cognitive impairment. The anti-cholinesterases block enzymes which break down acetylcholine, thus increasing its circulating levels.

Memantine works by controlling the response of NMDA receptors to the neurotransmitter glutamate. Glutamate is released when neurones and their support cells, astrocytes, are damaged, and glutamate itself causes further damage. Therefore, controlling the effect of glutamate helps protect neurones against further injury.

Usage

These drugs are not licensed for use in patients with purely vascular dementia, but can be used in those with mixed Alzheimer's and vascular disease. Rivastigmine is also licensed for use in dementia in Parkinson's disease.

There is currently no evidence to suggest that any of these drugs prevent the progression from Mild Cognitive Impairment (MCI) to dementia (Russ and Morling 2012).

Although they work in slightly different ways, there is little difference in effect between the anti-cholinesterases except for tolerability and mode of administration. Rivastigmine is available as a skin patch which may reduce gastrointestinal side effects and aid administration. Donepezil is usually the first choice due to cost. Memantine is licensed for severe Alzheimer's dementia, or moderate where anti-cholinesterases are not tolerated (NICE 2011).

Evidence base

These drugs have been consistently shown to be effective, with donepezil causing an average 1.2 point increase on Mini Mental State Examination after 24 weeks compared to placebo, and improvement in function. Similar results are seen with the other agents, with little statistically significant difference between them. (Birks 2006; Knowles 2006) Around 50% of patients prescribed donepezil see some improvement in their symptoms or functioning after 24 weeks. These medications' main benefit is in halting or slowing the clinical progression of dementia, rather than reversing the brain changes that have already occurred, and this should be emphasised to patients and caregivers. They can also delay the need for the patient to move into 24-hour care (Birks and Harvey 2006).

Side effects

The adverse effects usually subside within a few weeks, but some patients find these intolerable or persistent. These must be balanced against the likelihood of improvement or stabilisation in memory or functional impairment. The drugs are usually started at

Table 17.1 Summary of cholinesterase inhibitors and memantine

	Donepezil	*Rivastigmine*	*Galantamine*	*Memantine*
Indications	Mild to moderate Alzheimer's dementia	Mild to moderate Alzheimer's dementia, Mild to moderate dementia in Parkinson's disease	Mild to moderate Alzheimer's dementia	Moderate to severe Alzheimer's dementia
Usual maintenance dose	10mg once daily	3–6mg twice daily Patch available	16–24mg daily (modified release or divided doses)	20mg once daily
Most common side effects	Headache, appetite loss, dizziness, nausea, vomiting, diarrhoea, sleep disturbance	Headache, appetite loss, dizziness, nausea, vomiting, diarrhoea, sleep disturbance	Headache, appetite loss, dizziness, nausea, vomiting, diarrhoea, sleep disturbance	(These are less common than anti-cholinesterase side effects) Tiredness, dizziness, constipation, headache, shortness of breath
Rarer but important side effects	Slow pulse, seizures, urinary retention	Slow pulse, seizures, urinary retention	Slow pulse, seizures, urinary retention	Hallucinations, confusion, vomiting

Source: (BNF 2016).

low doses and gradually increased over several weeks, with the aim of minimising side effects.

Monitoring of weight and pulse is usually recommended for the initial period of treatment. It is also important, before starting an anti-cholinesterase, to address any concordance issues, such as arranging for a compliance aid (Anderson and Woodburn 2010).

Follow up and further prescribing options

It is recommended that cognition be tested around three months into a course of treatment. If there is no apparent benefit then the drug should be stopped. If there is a significant deterioration after stopping treatment, then most clinicians would take a pragmatic approach and consider re-starting it (BNF 2016).

There is only weak evidence to suggest that combining memantine and an anti-cholinesterase may help in moderate to severe Alzheimer's disease (Schmidt et al. 2015).

Drug treatment of Dementia with Lewy Bodies (DLB)

Anti-cholinesterases appear to give more benefit in DLB than Alzheimer's dementia (Rolinski et al. 2012) and patients with hallucinations may show increased benefit (McKeith et al. 2004). Abrupt withdrawal of anti-cholinesterases may lead to rebound worsening of BPSD (Minett et al. 2003). If a patient has responded they should continue on treatment and if the treatment must be discontinued, this should be done slowly. Memantine may be of modest benefit, but perhaps better used in combination with anti-cholinesterases in DLB (Emre et al. 2010).

Parkinson's disease-like symptoms occur in the majority of patients with DLB and it is a major cause of functional impairment. Guidance suggests these physical symptoms should be treated in the same way as Parkinson's disease. However anti-Parkinson's medications can worsen psychiatric symptoms in DLB and therefore caution is necessary (Goldman et al. 2008). Patients with DLB are often exquisitely sensitive to antipsychotics and these should therefore only be used when absolutely necessary (McKeith et al. 2005). Quetiapine has been recommended for psychotic symptoms in dementia with Parkinsonism but appears to be unhelpful (Kurlan et al. 2007). Low dose Clonazepam, Melatonin and Quetiapine may be helpful for REM sleep behaviour disorder (Aurora et al. 2010; Briggs et al. 2016).

Vascular dementia

Studies have shown some small statistically significant benefits from treatment with anti-cholinesterases but the magnitude of benefit is thought unlikely to be clinically significant (O'Brien and Thomas 2015).

Alternative treatments

There are various alternative treatments, such as ginseng and gingko biloba that are sometimes marketed as improving memory. However, there is no robust evidence to support their use in preventing dementia (Birks and Grimley Evans 2009; Geng et al. 2010). It is also worth noting that although such treatments are often described as "natural" they do have active ingredients with potential adverse effects and interactions with prescribed medications.

Potential drug developments

No new drugs for dementia have been licensed since 2002. Internationally, there were 413 trials of dementia drugs between 2002 and 2012, of which 99.6% failed to lead to new treatments (Cummings et al. 2014). Unfortunately, promising early phase trial results are often well-publicised in the media, unrealistically raising the hopes of patients and their carers. The drug development process from these initial stages takes many years.

It is thought that the deposition of amyloid in plaques in the brain may play a key role in leading to the neuronal damage which is the hallmark of Alzheimer's dementia. However one of the problems facing researchers and drug developers is that amyloid deposition predates the onset of clinical dementia by ten to 15 years, and some individuals with high levels of amyloid deposition may indeed never develop dementia (Riley et al. 2002). Drugs targeting the chemical pathways leading to amyloid deposition have shown no benefit in the treatment of dementia. New studies are using advanced imaging techniques to assess levels of amyloid deposition in people with early cognitive decline. It may then be possible for them to enter pilot studies to see if immunotherapy can prevent them from developing dementia (Briggs et al. 2016). In the event of future trials being successful, the use of disease-modifying treatments very early in the disease course would need health services to be redesigned (Ritchie et al. 2017).

There is a new emphasis on designing trials where the participants are healthy but have risk factors for dementia (for example, a family history) in order to test new drugs on these people at the very early stages of pathology developing (Ritchie et al. 2016). Other researchers are turning their focus towards preventing dementia by investigating and promoting lifestyle interventions in middle age (Livingston et al. 2017).

Notes

1　http://www.cochrane.org/.
2　http://www.alltrials.net/.

References

Alzheimer's Research UK. (2015) *Defeat dementia: the evidence and a vision for action*. Cambridge: Alzheimer's Research.

Anderson, N. and Woodburn, K. (2010) *Chapter 22, Old-age Psychiatry in Companion to Psychiatric Studies*. United Kingdom: Elsevier Health Sciences.

Aurora, R. N., Zak, R. S., Maganti, R. K., Auerbach, S. H., Casey, K. R., Chowdhuri, S., Karippot, A., Ramar, K., Kristo, D. A., Morgenthaler, T. I. and American Academy Of Sleep Medicine. (2010) "Best practice guide for the treatment of REM sleep behavior disorder (RBD)." *Journal of Clinical Sleep Medicine*, 6: 85–95.

Banerjee, S. (2009) *The use of antipsychotic medication for people with dementia: Time for action*. London: Department of Health.

Banerjee, S., Hellier, J., Dewey, M., Romeo, R., Ballard, C., Baldwin, R., Bentham, P., Fox, C., Holmes, C. and Katona, C. (2011) "Sertraline or mirtazapine for depression in dementia (HTA-SADD): a randomised, multicentre, double-blind, placebo-controlled trial." *The Lancet*, 378: 403–411.

Birks, J. and Grimley Evans, J. (2009) *Ginkgo biloba for cognitive impairment and dementia*. Oxford: The Cochrane Library. Available from: https://www.cochranelibrary.com/cdsr/doi/10.1002/14651858.CD003120.pub2/ful.

Birks, J. and Harvey, R. J. (2006) *Donepezil for dementia due to Alzheimer's disease*. The Oxford: The Cochrane Library. Available from: https://www.cochranelibrary.com/cdsr/doi/10.1002/14651858.CD001190/full .

Birks, J. S. (2006) *Cholinesterase inhibitors for Alzheimer's disease*. Oxford: The Cochrane Library. Available from: https://www.cochrane.org/CD005593/DEMENTIA_cholinesterase-inhibitors-cheis-donepezil-galantamine-and-rivastigmine-are-efficacious-mild-moderate.

BNF. (2016) *British National Formulary*. London: BMJ Group and Pharmaceutical Press. Available from: https://www.new.medicinescomplete.com/#/browse/bnf.

Briggs, R., Kennelly, S. P. and O'Neill, D. (2016) "Drug treatments in Alzheimer's disease." *Clinical Medicine*, 16: 247–253.

Corbett, A., Burns, A. and Ballard, C. (2014) "Don't use antipsychotics routinely to treat agitation and aggression in people with dementia." *British Medical Journal*, 349: g6420. DOI: doi:10.1136/bmj.g6420.

Corbett, A., Husebo, B., Malcangio, M., Staniland, A., Cohen-Mansfield, J., Aarsland, D. and Ballard, C. (2012) "Assessment and treatment of pain in people with dementia." *Nature Reviews Neurology*, 8: 264–274.

Cummings, J. L., Morstorf, T. and Zhong, K. (2014) "Alzheimer's disease drug-development pipeline: few candidates, frequent failures." *Alzheimer's research and therapy*, 6(1).

Emre, M., Tsolaki, M., Bonuccelli, U., Destée, A., Tolosa, E., Kutzelnigg, A., Ceballos-Baumann, A., Zdravkovic, S., Bladström, A. and Jones, R. (2010) "Memantine for patients with Parkinson's disease dementia or dementia with Lewy bodies: a randomised, double-blind, placebo-controlled trial." *The Lancet Neurology*, 9: 969–977.

Enache, D., Fereshtehnejad, S., Cermakova, P., Garcia-Ptacek, S., Kåreholt, I., Johnell, K., Religa, D., Jelic, V., Winblad, B. and Ballard, C. (2016) "Antidepressants and mortality risk in a dementia cohort–data from SveDem, the Swedish Dementia Registry." *European Psychiatry*, 33: S85.

Feldman, H., Gauthier, S., Hecker, J., Vellas, B., Xu, Y., Ieni, J. R. and Schwam, E. M. (2005) "Efficacy and safety of donepezil in patients with more severe Alzheimer's disease: a subgroup analysis from a randomized, placebo-controlled trial." *International Journal of Geriatric Psychiatry*, 20: 559–569.

Fleisher, A., Truran, D., Mai, J., Langbaum, J., Aisen, P., Cummings, J. L., Jack, C., Weiner, M., Thomas, R. and Schneider, L. (2011) "Chronic divalproex sodium use and brain atrophy in Alzheimer disease." *Neurology*, 77: 1263–1271.

Geng, J., Dong, J., Ni, H., Lee, M. S., Wu, T., Jiang, K., Wang, G., Zhou, A. L. and Malouf, R. (2010) *Ginseng for cognition*. Oxford: The Cochrane Library.

Glassock, R. J. and Winearls, C. (2009) "Ageing and the glomerular filtration rate: truths and consequences." *Transactions of the American Clinical and Climatological Association*, 120: 419.

Goldman, J. G., Goetz, C. G., Brandabur, M., Sanfilippo, M. and Stebbins, G. T. (2008) "Effects of dopaminergic medications on psychosis and motor function in dementia with Lewy bodies." *Movement Disorders*, 23: 2248–2250.

Gray, S. L., Anderson, M. L., Dublin, S., Hanlon, J. T., Hubbard, R., Walker, R., Yu, O., Crane, P. K. and Larson, E. B. (2015) "Cumulative use of strong anticholinergics and incident dementia: a prospective cohort study." *JAMA Internal Medicine*, 175: 401–407.

Guyatt, G. H., Oxman, A. D., Montori, V., Vist, G., Kunz, R., Brozek, J., Alonso-Coello, P., Djulbegovic, B., Atkins, D. and Falck-Ytter, Y. (2011) "GRADE guidelines: 5. Rating the quality of evidence-publication bias." *Journal of Clinical Epidemiology*, 64: 1277–1282.

Howard, R. J., Juszczak, E., Ballard, C. G., Bentham, P., Brown, R. G., Bullock, R., Burns, A. S., Holmes, C., Jacoby, R. and Johnson, T. (2007) "Donepezil for the treatment of agitation in Alzheimer's disease." *New England Journal of Medicine*, 357: 1382–1392.

Knowles, J. (2006) "Donepezil in Alzheimer's disease: an evidence-based review of its impact on clinical and economic outcomes." *Core Evidence*, 1: 195.

Konovalov, S., Muralee, S. and Tampi, R. R. (2008) "Anticonvulsants for the treatment of behavioral and psychological symptoms of dementia: a literature review." *International Psychogeriatrics*, 20: 293–308.

Kurlan, R., Cummings, J., Raman, R., Thal, L. (2007) "Quetiapine for agitation or psychosis in patients with dementia and parkinsonism." *Neurology*, 68: 1356–1363.

Lebert, F., Stekke, W., Hasenbroekx, C. and Pasquier, F. (2004) "Frontotemporal dementia: a randomised, controlled trial with trazodone." *Dementia and geriatric cognitive disorders*, 17: 355–359.

Livingston, G., Sommerlad, A., Orgeta, V., Costafreda, S. G., Huntley, J., Ames, D., Ballard, C., Banerjee, S., Burns, A. and Cohen-Mansfield, J. (2017) "Dementia prevention, intervention, and care." *The Lancet*, 390: 2673–2734.

Lonergan, E. and Luxenberg, J. (2009) *Valproate Preparations for Agitation in Dementia*. Oxford: The Cochrane Library.

McGuinness, B., Craig, D., Bullock, R. and Passmore, P. (2016) *Statins for the Prevention of Dementia*. Oxford: The Cochrane Library.

McKeith, I., Dickson, D. W., Lowe, J., Emre, M., O'Brien, J., Feldman, H., Cummings, J., Duda, J., Lippa, C. and Perry, E. (2005) "Diagnosis and management of dementia with Lewy bodies third report of the DLB consortium." *Neurology*, 65: 1863–1872.

McKeith, I. G., Wesnes, K. A., Perry, E. and Ferrara, R. (2004) "Hallucinations predict attentional improvements with rivastigmine in dementia with Lewy bodies." *Dementia and Geriatric Cognitive Disorders*, 18: 94–100.

Minett, T. S., Thomas, A., Wilkinson, L. M., Daniel, S. L., Sanders, J., Richardson, J., Littlewood, E., Myint, P., Newby, J. and McKeith, I. G. (2003) "What happens when donepezil is suddenly withdrawn? An open label trial in dementia with Lewy bodies and Parkinson's disease with dementia." *International Journal of Geriatric Psychiatry*, 18: 988–993.

NICE (2011) "Donepezil, galantamine, rivastigmine and memantine for the treatment of Alzheimer's disease." Technology appraisal guidance. Available from: https://www.nice.org.uk/Guidance/TA217.

O'Brien, J. T. and Thomas, A. (2015) "Vascular dementia." *The Lancet*, 386: 1698–1706.

O'Mahony, D., O'Sullivan, D., Byrne, S., O'Connor, M. N., Ryan, C. and Gallagher, P. (2014) "STOPP/START criteria for potentially inappropriate prescribing in older people: version 2." *Age and ageing*, 44(2): 213–218. doi:10.1093/ageing/afu145.

Richardson, K., Fox, C., Maidment, I., Steel, N., Loke, Y. K., Arthur, A., Myint, P. K., Grossi, C. M., Mattishent, K., Bennett, K., Campbell, N. L., Boustani, M., Robinson, L., Brayne, C., Matthews, F. E. and Savva, G. M. (2018) "Anticholinergic drugs and risk of dementia: case-control study." *British Medical Journal*, 361: k1315.

Riley, K. P., Snowdon, D. A. and Markesbery, W. R. (2002) "Alzheimer's neurofibrillary pathology and the spectrum of cognitive function: findings from the Nun Study." *Annals of Neurology*, 51: 567–577.

Ritchie, C. W., Molinuevo, J. L., Truyen, L., Satlin, A., Van Der Geyten, S. and Lovestone, S. (2016) "Development of interventions for the secondary prevention of Alzheimer's dementia: the European Prevention of Alzheimer's Dementia (EPAD) project." *The Lancet Psychiatry*, 3: 179–186.

Ritchie, C. W., Russ, T. C., Banerjee, S., Barber, B., Boaden, A., Fox, N. C., Holmes, C., Isaacs, J. D., Leroi, I., Lovestone, S., Norton, M., O'Brien, J., Pearson, J., Perry, R., Pickett, J., Waldman, A. D., Wong, W. L., Rossor, M. N. and Burns, A. (2017) "The Edinburgh Consensus: preparing for the advent of disease-modifying therapies for Alzheimer's disease." *Alzheimer's Research and Therapy*, 9: 85.

Rolinski, M., Fox, C., Maidment, I. and McShane, R. (2012) "Cholinesterase inhibitors for dementia with Lewy bodies, Parkinson's disease dementia and cognitive impairment in Parkinson's Disease." Oxford: The Cochrane Library. Available from: https://www.cochrane.org/CD006504/DEMENTIA_cholinesterase-inhibitors-are-beneficial-for-people-with-parkinsons-disease-and-dementia.

Rouch, L., Cestac, P., Hanon, O., Cool, C., Helmer, C., Bouhanick, B., Chamontin, B., Dartigues, J.-F., Vellas, B. and Andrieu, S. (2015) "Antihypertensive drugs, prevention of cognitive decline and dementia: a systematic review of observational studies, randomized controlled trials and meta-analyses, with discussion of potential mechanisms." *CNS Drugs*, 29: 113–130.

Russ, T. C. and Morling, J. R. (2012) "Cholinesterase inhibitors for mild cognitive impairment." Oxford: The Cochrane Library. Available from: https://www.cochranelibrary.com/cdsr/doi/10.1002/14651858.CD009132.pub2/abstract

Schmidt, R., Hofer, E., Bouwman, F., Buerger, K., Cordonnier, C., Fladby, T., Galimberti, D., Georges, J., Heneka, M. and Hort, J. (2015) "Efns-Ens/Ean Guideline on concomitant use of cholinesterase inhibitors and memantine in moderate to severe Alzheimer's disease." *European Journal of Neurology*, 22: 889–898.

Seitz, D. P., Adunuri, N., Gill, S. S., Gruneir, A., Herrmann, N. and Rochon, P. (2011) "Antidepressants for agitation and psychosis in dementia." Oxford: The Cochrane Library. Available from: https://www.cochrane.org/CD008191/DEMENTIA_antidepressants-for-agitation-and-psychosis-in-dementia.

Suh, D.-C., Arcona, S., Thomas, S. K., Powers, C., Rabinowicz, A. L., Shin, H. and Mirski, D. (2004) "Risk of antipsychotic drug use in patients with Alzheimer's disease treated with rivastigmine." *Drugs and Aging*, 21: 395–403.

Tariot, P. N., Solomon, P., Morris, J., Kershaw, P., Lilienfeld, S. and Ding, C. (2000) "A 5-month, randomized, placebo-controlled trial of galantamine in AD." *Neurology*, 54: 2269–2276.

Van der Spek, K., Koopmans, R. T., Smalbrugge, M., Nelissen-Vrancken, M. H., Wetzels, R. B., Smeets, C. H., De Vries, E., Teerenstra, S., Zuidema, S. U. and Gerritsen, D. L. (2018) "The effect of biannual medication reviews on the appropriateness of psychotropic drug use for neuropsychiatric symptoms in patients with dementia: a randomised controlled trial." *Age and Ageing*, 47: 430–437.

Young, J., Murthy, L., Westby, M., Akunne, A. and O'Mahony, R. (2010) "Diagnosis, prevention, and management of delirium: summary of NICE guidance." *British Medical Journal*, 341: c3704.

Further reading

Ritchie, C. W., Molinuevo, J. L., Truyen, L., Satlin, A., Van Der Geyten, S. and Lovestone, S. (2016) "Development of interventions for the secondary prevention of Alzheimer's dementia: the European Prevention of Alzheimer's Dementia (EPAD) project." *The Lancet Psychiatry*, 3: 179–186.

18 Delirium

Rekha Hegde and Ajay Macharouthu

Introduction

Delirium and dementia are disorders of cognitive function and are associated with adverse health outcomes. They are inextricably linked and it is difficult to talk about one without the other. Dementia is a risk factor for developing delirium (Ahmed et al. 2014). Delirium is associated with the extremes of age: its prevalence increases with age. Innovations in healthcare around the world have had a significant impact on longevity, thereby changing the contours of the population pyramid, as well as of these disorders. There are various strategic drivers aimed at improving delirium and dementia care, including The National Dementia Strategy (Scottish Government 2013), Care of older people in hospital standards (Healthcare Improvement Scotland 2015a), Older people in hospital inspections (Healthcare Improvement Scotland 2015b) and Think Delirium (Healthcare Improvement Scotland 2016), which are instrumental in meeting this demographic challenge.

Current knowledge

The word "delirium" was first used as a medical term as early as the first century AD to describe mental disorders occurring during fever or head trauma. A diverse range of inappropriate terms have since emerged to describe delirium, including "acute confusional state", "acute brain syndrome", "acute cerebral insufficiency" and "toxic–metabolic encephalopathy". However it is felt that the term "delirium" should be used as a standard term for this syndrome with important outcomes.

Delirium is a serious acute neuropsychiatric condition affecting mainly older people. It is a syndrome characterised by acute onset with a fluctuating change in mental status with inattention, perceptual disturbances, disorganised thinking, sleep disturbance and altered level of consciousness.

How does it present?

The clinical presentation of delirium can be broadly classified into three sub-types, hyperactive and hypoactive (Liptzin and Levkoff 1992) and a third subtype, mixed delirium (O'Keeffe and Lavan 1999). Hyperactive delirium is characterised by heightened arousal, restlessness, agitation and aggression. A hypoactive delirium is characterised by sleepiness, disengagement in daily activities and being quiet and withdrawn, all of which are sometimes mistaken as symptoms of depression. Mixed delirium is characterised by a presentation which fluctuates between the two subtypes. Delirium without agitation predominantly occurs in greater than 50% of patients with hypoactive and mixed delirium, which are under diagnosed or undiagnosed. Some studies have reported that hypoactive delirium is often associated with worse outcome (Kiely et al. 2007), thereby highlighting the need for increased vigilance for this subtype.

The differential diagnosis of delirium includes dementia and other functional psychiatric disorders. The differences between delirium, dementia and depression are delineated in Table 18.1. Typically, delirium presents with an abrupt presentation of a fluctuating course with clouding of consciousness in comparison to dementia where the person is alert with a gradual and progressive course over a period of six months. Dementia of Lewy bodies is an exception where the clinical symptoms would mirror delirium with a rapid onset, thereby posing a diagnostic challenge. Depressive disorder can further confuse the diagnosis with a "pseudo-dementia" picture and it's important to note that the person is alert with pervasive low mood over a period of two weeks with a lack of interest and energy, which is reflected in poor scores on cognitive testing. A good collateral history will help determine what the most likely diagnosis is.

It is important to remember that in a vulnerable frail elderly person, a minor precipitant such as catheterisation or constipation can increase the risk of delirium.

The physiology of delirium can be understood when a stressor (pain/constipation/infection/dehydration) causes activation of the normal stress response, engaging the hypo-thalamic-pituitary axis that results in a pro-inflammatory response with the release of cortisol and then IL-2–6/TNF/cytokines in the circulatory system (Rudolph et al. 2008) (see Figure 18.2). At the extremes of age the blood brain barrier's efficiency is compromised thus allowing these pro-inflammatory chemicals access to the brain. Peripherally secreted cytokines can provoke exaggerated responses from microglia, thereby causing severe inflammation in the brain (Dilger and Johnson 2008; Dunn 2006). It is thought that people with dementia have pathological damage to their neurones as well as structural changes, which renders them vulnerable to the effects of these cytokines disrupting normal function and resulting in abnormal neurotransmitter release (Burns et al. 2004).

Pro-inflammatory cytokines can substantially affect the synthesis or release of neurotransmitters such as acetylcholine, dopamine, norepinephrine and 5-HT, thereby disrupting neuronal communication (Dilger andJohnson 2008; Dunn 2006). Given the role that

Table 18.1 Differential diagnosis of delirium

	Delirium	*Dementia*	*Depression*
Onset	Acute	Insidious	Variable
Duration	Days to weeks	Months to years (6 months)	Two weeks
Course	Fluctuating	Slowly progressive	Diurnal variation (worse in morning, improves during day)
Consciousness	Impaired, fluctuates	Clear until late in the course of illness	Unimpaired
Attention and memory	Inattentive, poor memory	Poor memory with inattention	Difficulty concentrating; memory intact
Affect	Variable	Variable	Depressed; loss of interest and pleasure

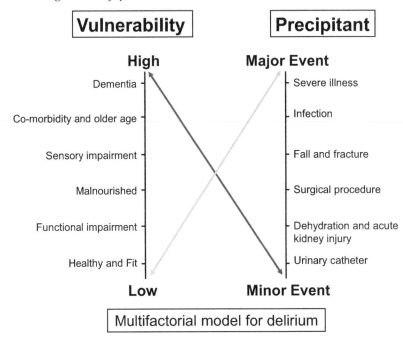

| Vulnerability | Precipitant |

High   **Major Event**

Dementia — / .... \ — Severe illness

Co-morbidity and older age — — Infection

Sensory impairment — — Fall and fracture

Malnourished — — Surgical procedure

Functional impairment — — Dehydration and acute kidney injury

Healthy and Fit — — Urinary catheter

Low   **Minor Event**

| Multifactorial model for delirium |

Figure 18.1 Multifactorial model of delirium
Source: Adapted from Jackson et al. (2017).

acetylcholine plays in short term memory and orientation it is not surprising that there are relative deficits in the amount of acetylcholine released in delirious patients. However, other studies have not found a clear association between serum anti-cholinergic activity and delirium. Just as there is an imbalance between acetylcholine and dopamine, so too is there a relative excess of the excitatory neurotransmitter glutamate and a relative deficit of the inhibitory neurotransmitter GABA (Gaudreau and Gagnon 2005).

This imbalance translates to the clinical picture we see. The relative excess of dopamine accounts for the psychotic symptoms and paranoia that can often be experienced by those with hyperactive delirium. Anti-parkinsonian drugs can cause delirium, and dopamine antagonists such as haloperidol are effective in controlling the symptoms of delirium (Young, 1997).

How common is it?

The prevalence of delirium in the community is difficult to estimate. Community based point prevalence of delirium is between 0.63% and 1.09%. A meta-analysis reported a pooled prevalence of 0.72 % in people aged 65 years and over (Davis et al. 2013). In care homes the prevalence is much higher, ranging from 6.5% to 70.3% de Lange et al. 2013).

Delirium is common among older people in hospital and those admitted to hospital with delirium are traditionally described as prevalent delirium or community acquired delirium. Prevalent delirium in emergency departments is reported to be between 8% and 10% (Han et al. 2010). A systematic review reported prevalence among older people admitted to hospital of between 10% and 31% (Siddiqui et al. 2006).

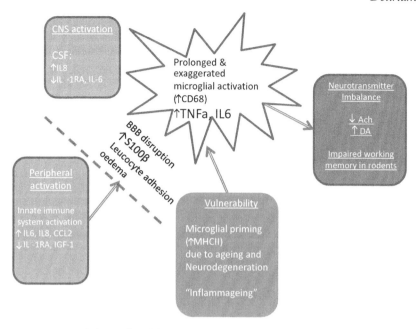

Figure 18.2 Patho-physiology of delirium
Source: Adapted from Jackson et al. (2017).

Incident delirium is seen in people already admitted to hospital and thereby representing hospital acquired delirium. A systematic review of studies (Davis et al 2013; de Lange et al. 2013; Han et al. 2010; Siddiqui et al. 2006) reports delirium incidence ranging from 3% to 25% during the in-patient stay. Incident delirium is common after surgical procedures. Incidence is up to 46% in cardiac surgery, 50% in non-cardiac surgery and 51% in orthopaedic surgery. In intensive care settings, again there is a wide reported prevalence and incidence with a reported range of 20%–80%.

Added knowledge

Why is delirium important when thinking about people with dementia?

Delirium is associated with adverse clinical outcomes: increased mortality; increased length of hospital stay; increased rates of institutionalisation; and development of dementia (Siddiqui et al. 2006; Witlox et al. 2010). The adverse outcomes described cause significant morbidity for both the patient and their carers and thus have significant health economy cost (Leslie et al. 2008). Dementia is a risk factor for developing delirium (Ahmed et al. 2014). Delirium superimposed on dementia accounts for up to 65% of all older people with delirium in hospital (Fick et al. 2002). Delirium can worsen already existing dementia (Fong et al, 2012) and is an independent risk factor for novel incident dementia (Davis et al. 2012).

The costs of delirium to the individual with dementia are high, and the healthcare costs are significant. People with dementia are three to five times more likely to develop a delirium than those without dementia and having an episode of delirium increases the risk of developing dementia by eight times (Davis et al. 2012). Delirium is also

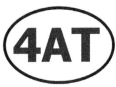

4AT

Assessment test
for delirium &
cognitive impairment

Patient name:

Date of birth:

Patient number:

Date: Time:

Tester:

CIRCLE

[1] ALERTNESS

This includes patients who may be markedly drowsy (eg. difficult to rouse and/or obviously sleepy during assessment) or agitated/hyperactive. Observe the patient. If asleep, attempt to wake with speech or gentle touch on shoulder. Ask the patient to state their name and address to assist rating.

Normal (fully alert, but not agitated, throughout assessment)	0
Mild sleepiness for <10 seconds after waking, then normal	0
Clearly abnormal	4

[2] AMT4

Age, date of birth, place (name of the hospital or building), current year.

No mistakes	0
1 mistake	1
2 or more mistakes/untestable	2

[3] ATTENTION

Ask the patient: "Please tell me the months of the year in backwards order, starting at December."
To assist initial understanding one prompt of "what is the month before December?" is permitted.

Months of the year backwards

Achieves 7 months or more correctly	0
Starts but scores <7 months / refuses to start	1
Untestable (cannot start because unwell, drowsy, inattentive)	2

[4] ACUTE CHANGE OR FLUCTUATING COURSE

Evidence of significant change or fluctuation in: alertness, cognition, other mental function (eg. paranoia, hallucinations) arising over the last 2 weeks and still evident in last 24hrs

No	0
Yes	4

---

4 or above: possible delirium +/- cognitive impairment
1-3: possible cognitive impairment
0: delirium or severe cognitive impairment unlikely (but delirium still possible if [4] information incomplete)

4AT SCORE [ ]

Figure 18.3 4AT test
Source: Permission granted by Prof A. MacLullich.

Delirium Identification

Expect it in vulnerable brain

People with dementia are at high risk in hospital, including people with previous delirium. Plan and protect vulnerable people

Speak to family and carers

They will provide you with collateral history to investigate an acute change. Always speak to someone who knows the person

Use identification tool

Use the 4AT to help you identify delirium in those at risk in your care

Hyperactive delirium

Can be present on admission or develop in hospital. Easier to spot due to agitated behaviour, confusion and hallucinations always?

Early recognition

For every 48 hours delirium is undetected, mortality increases by 11%

Hypoactive delirium*

Have concern for a newly sleepy, drowsy person with acute illness presenting or developing in hospital. High risk of aspiration and mortality

*Remember delirium can also be mixed hyperactive and hypoactive, look for causes

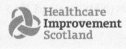

SCOTTISH
DELIRIUM
ASSOCIATION

Figure 18.4 Delirium identification
Source: Adapted from HIS.

Table 18.2 Risk factors for delirium

Risk factors for delirium		Precipitating factors for delirium	
Demographics	**Decreased intake**	**Drugs**	**Illness**
Older age	Dehydration	Sedatives, Narcotics,	Infection
Male	Malnutrition	anti-	Metabolic imbalance
Cognitive status	**Drugs**	Cholinergic	Hypoxia
Dementia	Polypharmacy	Polypharmacy	Shock
Cognitive	Anticholinergic	Alcohol or drug	Anaemia
Impairment	Alcohol abuse	withdrawal	Hypothermia
History of delirium	**Medical comorbidity**	**Environmental**	Dehydration
Depression	High severity of	Too much or too	Low serum albumin
Functional status	illness	little stimulation	Acid base imbalance
Functional	High level of	Use of physical	Fever
dependence	comorbidity	restraint	Severe illness
Immobility	Chronic renal or	Bladder catheter use	**Surgery**
Falls	hepatic impairment	Pain	Orthopaedic/cardiac
Poor activity level	**Disease**	Emotional distress	Non-cardiac
Sensory impairment	Stroke	Prolonged sleep	Duration of cardio-
Vision and hearing	Neurological disease	deprivation	Pulmonary bypass
	Metabolic imbalance	Multiple ward moves	
	Fracture/trauma		
	Terminal illness		
	HIV		

associated with worsening dementia severity (odds ratio 3.1, 95% confidence interval 1.5–6.3) as well as deterioration in global function score (odds ratio 2.8, 95% confidence interval 1.4–5.5) (Davis at al. 2012).

There is an acceptance now that delirium should be considered as a medical emergency until proven otherwise; mortality rates for patients admitted to hospital with delirium can range from 10% to 26% (Fong et al. 2009). Until recently it has not been given the same prominence as heart disease, stroke or pneumonia. As well as increased mortality rates, patients with delirium have an increased length of stay, and increased risk of institutional placement. There is a higher risk of hospital acquired complications such as pressure sores and falls (Inouye and Marcantonio 2007). Up to 60% of individuals suffer persistent cognitive impairment following delirium (Levkoff et al. 1992; Murray et al. 1993)

The cost implications to the NHS are huge. For example, an orthopaedics bed costs around £700 per day with an average length of stay being extra three to five days (MacLullich 2015). The indirect costs of delirium increasing disease burden of dementia is a significant challenge for the NHS, with an estimated 25% of acute beds occupied by people with dementia, rising to 40% or even higher in elderly care wards (NHS England 2015–16).

Where we can do things better

Improving detection

The incidence rates of delirium during a hospital stay are now recognised as a sign of quality of hospital care (Inouye et al. 1999). Good nursing care and proactive management of modifiable risk factors, such as dehydration, pain, constipation, sensory impairments and poor mobility can reduce incidence rates.

Delirium Risk Reduction

Sleep in hospital
Promote good environment for restful sleep

Sight and hearing
Helping people with sensory impairment by using glasses and hearing aids in hospital

Hydration
Ensure people at risk have adequate plan for hydration in hospital

Prolonged hospital stay
Work together to plan for discharge, avoiding prolonged stay

Identification
One in five people in acute hospitals can have delirium

Medication
Avoid high risk medication in people at risk of delirium. Think about pain

Promoting mobility and function
Design plan of care to promote mobility and function

Constipation
Optimise bowel health/function in those at risk

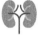

Renal function
Preserve renal function ensuring medicine reconciliation is carried out and hydration status is monitored in those at risk

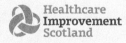

Healthcare **Improvement** Scotland

SCOTTISH **DELIRIUM** ASSOCIATION

Figure 18.5 Delirium risk-reduction
Source: Adapted from HIS.

The risk of developing delirium can be reduced in hospitals in one third of service users (Inouye et al. 1999; Marcantonio et al. 2001). Despite this, and its significant adverse outcomes, delirium detection rates remain low. For example, a study by Collins et al. (2010) of 710 acute elderly medical admissions found that the clinical teams did not pick up 72% of 110 delirium cases. Delirium is mis-diagnosed, detected late or missed in over 50% of cases across healthcare settings. In addition, dementia is thought to be an underlying condition in up to 50% of delirium in elderly patients and is known to be a potent predisposing factor for the development of delirium. Thus, improving delirium detection with the help of appropriate delirium screening tools such as a 4AT test (Bellelli et al. 2014) and acquiring corroborative history from appropriate carers is desirable.

The diagnosis of delirium is clinical. Recognition is improved by having a high level of clinical suspicion. No laboratory test can diagnose delirium. In about 10%–20% of patients, no cause is identified (Huang 2018). It is recognised that the cognitive effects of an episode of delirium can be persistent, thereby increasing the difficult to accurately diagnose the presence of dementia in this time period.

Practice recommendations

Looking at the predisposing factors a large proportion of patients admitted to hospital are at high risk of delirium. By embedding the use of screening tools in Accident and Emergency and Medical Assessment Units, the detection rate can be improved. The "Think Delirium" (Healthcare Improvement Scotland 2016) initiative developed by Healthcare Improvement Scotland (HIS) in coordination with the Scottish Delirium Association (SDA) uses the 4 AT screening tool and Time bundle (Healthcare Improvement Scotland 2016) proactively for frail elderly patients with hip fracture, severe illness and cognitive impairment and encourages active care focussing on hydration, orientation, pain, bowels, bladder, hearing and sight.

In trying to reduce rates of delirium and therefore dementia we also need to examine how this group of patients is currently managed in a general hospital setting. It is easy to see that the existing hospital flow is not designed to optimally manage delirious patients. A patient journey within a hospital typically results in a number of ward moves, which in itself is a cause for delirium. Frequent nursing shifts and busy wards are unhelpful for delirious patients and premature discharge planning in itself can result in failed discharges and readmissions.

1   Lack of corroborative history
2   Assume cognitive impairment is long-standing
3   No assessment of cognitive functions
4   Not talking to nurses, especially the night staff
5   Not involving families
6   If patient is withdrawn, starting an antidepressant
7   If patient is distressed, prescribing a benzodiazepine

Figure 18.6 Delirium diagnosis: Missed opportunities

Delirium Management

Educate people and their families

Help families and carers understand what is happening. Help them to be involved in the care of their loved ones. It is important for recognition of potential future episodes

Look for triggers

By taking a thorough history first treat the cause or causes. Think medication change, addition or withdrawal, pain, dehydration, electrolyte disturbance, sepsis, constipation and retention

Use management tool

Ensure safety by using a systematic approach. The TIME Bundle will reduce variation in care.
THINK, INVESTIGATE, MANAGE, ENGAGE & EXPLAIN

Think about follow up

It is important to write DELIRIUM in the notes, on the discharge letter and refer to appropriate follow-up ensuring safe transition of care. Connect the chain of people caring for the person

It can be fatal

For every FIVE people diagnosed with delirium ONE will be dead within a month

Reduce risk of falling

People with delirium are at great risk of falling. Always consider your plan to reduce in both care domains. 68% of people who fall in hospital have cognitive impairment

Think about Stress and Distress

Remember that people with dementia are at high risk of developing delirium

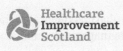
Healthcare
Improvement
Scotland

SCOTTISH
DELIRIUM
ASSOCIATION

Figure 18.7 Delirium management
Source: Adapted from HIS.

Given that delirium is highly prevalent in community and nursing homes, it is imperative that this group is appropriately managed prior to hospital admission. Nursing homes are ill equipped in managing delirium and an integrated approach such as the "hospital at home" work stream would be a way forward. This would redefine care in nursing homes with IV fluids and antibiotics being administered by skilled staff with adequate support and supervision. The Stop Delirium! Intervention (Siddiqui 2011) an enhanced educational package for care home staff (incorporating strategies to change practice, such as adapting to the local context, interactive teaching methods, promoting ownership and championing) is a helpful strategy. This approach to delirium risk reduction is well supported by the research literature from hospital settings and is consistent with NICE guidelines (NICE 2010).

How to approach the management of a delirious patient

Delirium management includes non-pharmacological and pharmacological strategies, detailed in Figures 18.7 and 18.8. Early identification with appropriate screening instruments and the TIME management tool with risk reduction strategies is the key to successful management of delirium. It is important to engage with the family and educate them about Delirium. Carers should be involved as partners in delirium care and the Delirium information leaflet (Healthcare Improvement Scotland 2016) goes a long away in improving the understanding about this complex disorder.

- Reduce sensory impairment
- Ensure adequate light
- Make environment clutter free
- Re-orientation strategies - Use clocks with time and date, calendars
- Well positioned signs
- Use familiar objects, family and friends
- Consistency in staff
- Ambient room temperature
- Make sure not too noisy or busy or quiet.
- Use a single side room
- Consider one to one nursing
- Allow movement/facilitate mobility
- Address simple issues like pain, constipation, dehydration, hunger.
- Use music that the person likes, to sooth

Figure 18.8 Non pharmacological interventions in delirium

Consider non-pharmacological strategies before pharmacological strategies in dealing with stress and distress. The SDA's Delirium management summary pathway flowchart (Figure 18.7) is very helpful in this regard (www.scottishdeliriumassociation.com). Assessments of capacity should be incorporated where appropriate with relevant adults with incapacity/mental capacity legislation being considered.

Pharmacological strategies include medication reconciliation thereby appropriately stopping and reducing medications that have the potential to increase the risk of developing delirium. Extremely distressed patients may benefit from brief intervention with antipsychotic medication such as Haloperidol in appropriate doses for a short period with daily reviews (NICE 2010). Benzodiazepines have a

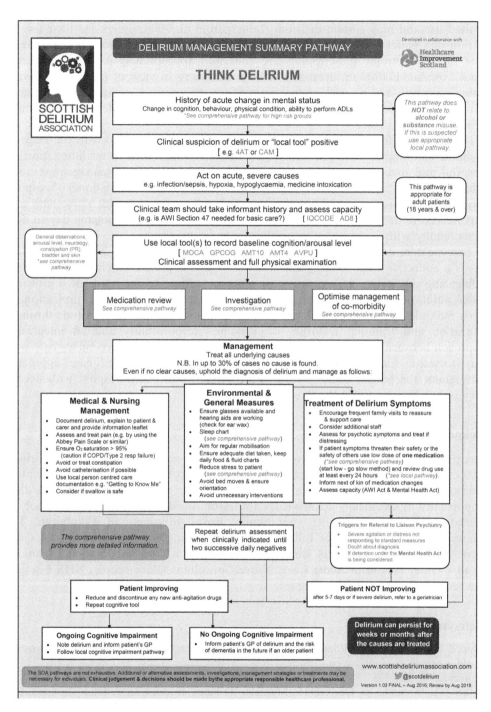

Figure 18.9 Delirium management–Summary pathway
Source: Adapted from SDA.

limited use and may sustain delirium (Lonergan et al. 2009) except for their use in Parkinson's patients where antipsychotics are used only with caution. It's important that the psychotropic prescriptions are addressed appropriately prior to discharge from hospital. Follow up arrangements are necessary in view of the risk of developing dementia and as well as the traumatic experiences. A comprehensive cognitive assessment post-discharge can further identify new cases of dementia that may otherwise go unnoticed.

Hospital care for a distressed patient could be further improved with the help of a shared care approach in the form of a "delirium ward" with better integration of hospital and mental health professionals. This allows proactive management, and rehabilitation by a multidisciplinary team consisting of a occupational therapist, physiotherapist, social worker, geriatric nurse and a mental health nurse who are experienced in delirium care, working on a recovery model in enhancing day to day functionality with a view to a successful discharge planning.

To conclude, delirium remains a major unmet medical need in healthcare, which needs a collective responsibility and a collaborative approach amongst clinicians in influencing qualitative and quantitative outcomes. Meeting the needs of a growing older adult population requires a cultural shift amongst healthcare professionals from multiple disciplines in addressing various issues with the right attitude through education and training. Delirium is everyone's responsibility and an integrated approach between health and social care as well as primary and secondary care is a way forward. Future innovation should be based on a shared care approach throughout the patient journey from the community into the hospital with necessary ownership embraced by all clinicians involved.

Acknowledgements

We gratefully acknowledge the work on delirium associated with Scottish Delirium Association (SDA) and Healthcare Improvement Scotland (HIS) and the related delirium pathways that were shared accordingly. We would also like to take this opportunity to specifically acknowledge Professor Alasdair MacLullich, Professor of Geriatric Medicine, Honorary consultant, Royal Infirmary of Edinburgh, Dr Thomas Jackson, Institute of Inflammation and Ageing, Clinician Scientist in Geriatric Medicine, University of Birmingham and Karen Goudie – National Clinical Lead – Older Person in Acute Care, Nurse Consultant Older people, NHS Fife for the resources utilised in this chapter.

References

Ahmed, S., Leurent, B. and Sampson, E.L. (2014) "Risk factors for incident delirium among older people in acute hospital medical units: a systematic review and meta-analysis." *Age Ageing*, 43: 326–333.

Bellelli, G., Morandi, A., Davis, D.H., Mazzola, P., Turco, R., Gentile, S., Ryan, T., Cash, H., Guerini, F., Torpilliesi, T., Del Santo, F., Trabucchi, M., Annoni, G., MacLullich, A.M.

(2014) "Validation of the 4AT, a new instrument for rapid delirium screening: a study in 234 hospitalised older people." *Age and Ageing*, 43: 496–502.

Burns, A., Gallagley, A. and Byrne, J. (2004) "Delirium." *Journal of Neurosurgery and Psychiatry*, 75(3): 362–367.

Collins, N., Blanchard, M., Tookman, A. and Sampson, E. (2010) "Detection of delirium in the acute hospital." *Age and Ageing*, 39(1): 131–135.

Davis, D.H., Muniz Terrera, G., Keage, H., Rahkonen, T., Oinas, M., Matthews, F.E., Cunningham, C., Polvikoski, T., Sulkava, R., MacLullich, A.M. and Brayne, C. (2012) "Delirium is a strong risk factor for dementia in the oldest-old: a population-based cohort study." *Brain*, 135: 2809–2816. doi:10.1093/brain/aws190.

De Lange, E., Verhaak, P.F.M. and Van Der Meer, K. (2013) "Prevalence, presentation and prognosis of delirium in older people in the population, at home and in long term care: a review." *International Journal of Geriatric Psychiatry*, 28: 127–134.

Department of Health. (2010) "Improving the Quality of care for people with Dementia in General Hospitals." Available from: http://www.hospitaldr.co.uk/Dementia%20care_EN_1.pdf.

Dilger, R.N. and Johnson, R.W. (2008) "Aging, microglial cell priming, and the discordant central inflammatory response to signals from the peripheral immune system." *Journal of Leukocyte Biology*, 84(4): 932–939.

Dunn, A.J. (2006) "Effects of cytokines and infections on brain neurochemistry." *Clinical Neuroscience Research*, 6(1–2): 52–68.

Fick, D.M., Agostini, J.V. and Inouye, S.K. (2002) "Delirium superimposed on dementia: a systematic review." *Journal of the American Geriatric Society*, 50: 1723–1732.

Fong, T., Tulebaev, S. and Inouye, S. (2009) "Delirium in elderly adults: diagnosis, prevention and treatment." *Nature Reviews Neurology*, 5(4): 210–220. doi:10.1038/nrneurol.2009.24.

Fong, T.G., Jones, R.N., Marcantonio, E.R., Tommet, D., Gross, A.L., Habtemariam, D., Schmitt, E. and Yap, L. (2012) "Adverse outcomes after hospitalization and delirium in persons with Alzheimer Disease." *Annual Internal Medicine*, 156: 848–856.

Gaudreau, J.D. and Gagnon, P. (2005) "Psychotogenic drugs and delirium pathogenesis: the central role of the thalamus." *Medical Hypotheses*, 64(3): 471–475.

Han, J.H., Wilson, A. and Ely, E.W. (2010) "Delirium in the older emergency department patient: a quiet epidemic." *Emergency Medicine Clinics of North America*, 28: 611–631.

Healthcare Improvement Scotland. (2015a) "Care of older people in hospital standards." Available from: http://www.healthcareimprovementscotland.org/our_work/person-centred_care/resources/opah_standards.aspx.

Healthcare Improvement Scotland. (2015b) "Inspecting the care of older people in acute hospitals." Available from: http://www.healthcareimprovementscotland.org/our_work/person-centred_care/resources/opah_standards.aspx.

Healthcare Improvement Scotland. (2016) "Improving the care for older people – Delirium Toolkit." Available from: http://www.healthcareimprovementscotland.org/our_work/person-centred_care/opac_improvement_programme/delirium_toolkit.aspx.

Huang, J. (2018) "Delirium Merck Manual." Available from: http://www.msdmanuals.com/en-gb/professional/neurologic-disorders/delirium-and-dementia/delirium#v1036474.

Inouye, S. and Marcantonio, E. (2007) "Delirium." (Eds) in Growdon, J. and Rossor, M. *The Dementias*. Philadelphia: Butterworth-Heinemann Elsevier. 285–312.

Inouye, S.K., Schlesinger, M.J. and Lydon, T.J. (1999) "Delirium: a symptom of how hospital care is failing older persons and a window to improve quality of hospital care." *American Journal of Medicine*, 106: 565–573.

Inouye, S.K., Westendorp, R.G.J. and Saczynski, J.S. (2014) "Delirium in elderly people." *The Lancet*, 383: 911–922.

Jackson, T.A., Gladman, J.R.F., Harwood, R., MacLullich, A., Sampson, E., Sheehan, B. and Davis, D. (2017) "Challenges and opportunities in understanding dementia and delirium in the acute hospital." *PLoS Med*, 14(3): e1002247. doi:10.1371/journal.pmed.1002247.

Kiely, D.K., Jones, R.N., Bergmann, M.A. and Marcantonio, E.R. (2007) "Association between psychomotor activity delirium subtypes and mortality among newly admitted postacute facility patients." *Journals of Gerontology Series A-Biological Sciences and Medical Sciences*, 62: 174–179.

Leslie, D.L., Marcantonio, E.R., Zhang, Y., Leo-Summers, L. and Inouye, S.K. (2008) "One-year health care costs associated with delirium in the elderly population." *Archives of Internal Medicine*, 168: 27–32.

Levkoff, S.E., Evans, D.A., Liptzin, B., Cleary, P.D., Lipsitz, L.A., Wetle, T.T., Reilly, C.H., Pilgrim, D.M., Schor, J. and Rowe, J. (1992) "Delirium. The occurrence and persistence of symptoms among elderly hospitalized patients." *Archives of Internal Medicine*, 152(2): 334–340.

Liptzin, B. and Levkoff, S.E. (1992) "An empirical study of delirium subtypes." *British Journal of Psychiatry*, 161: 843–845.

Lonergan, E., Luxenberg, J., Areosa Sastre, A. and Wyller, T.B. (2009) "Benzodiazepines for delirium." *Cochrane Database Syst Rev.* 2009 Jan 21;(1): CD006379. DOI: 10.1002/14651858. CD006379.pub2.

MacLullich, A. (2015) "NHS should view delirium as a medical emergency, experts warn." *Herald Scotland.* Available from: http://www.heraldscotland.com/news/13413907.NHS_should_view_delirium_as_a_medical_emergency__experts_warn/.

Marcantonio, E.R., Flacker, J.M., Wright, R.J. and Resnick, N.M. (2001) "Reducing delirium after hip fracture: a randomized trial." *Journal of the American Geriatric Society*, 49: 516–522.

Murray, A.M, Levkoff, S., Wetle, T., Beckett, L., Cleary, P., Schor, J., Lipsitz, L., Rowe, J., and Evans, D. (1993) "Acute delirium and functional decline in the hospitalized elderly patient." *Journal of Gerontology*, 48: M181–M186.

National Institute for Health and Clinical Excellence. (2010) "Delirium: prevention, diagnosis and management clinical guideline (CG103)." London, National Institute for Health and Clinical Excellence.

NHS England. (2015–16) "Commission for Quality and Innovation Guidance." Available from: https://www.england.nhs.uk/wp-content/uploads/2015/03/9-cquin-guid-2015-16.pdf.

O'Keeffe, S.T. and Lavan, J.N. (1999) "Clinical significance of delirium subtypes in older people." *Age and Ageing*, 28: 115–119.

Rudolph, J.L., Ramlawi, B., Kuchel, G.A., McElhaney, J.E., Xie, D., Sellke, F.W., Khabbaz, K. and Marcantonio, E.R. (2008) "Chemokines are associated with delirium after cardiac surgery." *The Journals of Gerontology. Series A, Biological Sciences and Medical Sciences*, 63(2): 184–189.

Scottish Government. (2013–16) "Scotland's National Dementia Strategy." Available from: http://www.gov.scot/Topics/Health/Services/Mental-Health/Dementia/DementiaStrategy1316.

Siddiqi, N. (2011) "Stop Delirium! A complex intervention to prevent." *Age and Ageing*, 40(1): 90–98. doi:10.1093/ageing/afq126.

Siddiqi, N., House, A.O. and Holmes, J.D. (2006) "Occurrence and outcome of delirium in medical in-patients: a systematic literature review." *Age and Ageing*, 35: 350–364.

Witlox, J., Eurelings, L.S., De Jonghe, J.F., Kalisvaart, K.J., Eikelenboom, P. and Van Gool, W.A. (2010) "Delirium in elderly patients and the risk of postdischarge mortality, institutionalization, and dementia: a meta-analysis." *Journal of the American Geriatric Association*, 304(4): 443–451. doi:10.1001/jama.2010.1013.

Young, B.K. (1997) "Neuropsychiatric adverse effects of antiparkinsonian drugs. Characteristics, evaluation and treatment." *Drugs and Ageing*, 10(5): 367–383.

Further reading

Scottish Delirium Association Guidelines. (2017) "Delirium Guidelines." Available from: http://www.scottishdeliriumassociation.com/guidelines–standards.html.

19 Younger person with dementia

Louise Ritchie

Although age is the main risk factor for dementia, around 5% of people diagnosed are under the age of 65. This is commonly referred to as Young or Early Onset Dementia. Individuals who receive a diagnosis of dementia at an earlier stage in their lives face a different set of circumstances than an individual who is diagnosed later in life. This includes still being in employment, having dependent children and having more financial commitments. Therefore, there is an argument that younger people with dementia have different care and support needs from people who are diagnosed with dementia in later life.

Thinking about society's expectation of the life course, it is clear that a person who is under the age of 65 is perceived as having a different role in society than someone who is over 65. The cut off age for young onset dementia being 65 is largely for social and economic reasons; in many western countries 65 is the standard age of retirement. According to Erikson's (1959) developmental theory of the lifespan, people between the ages of 40 and 65 are at the peak of their responsibility in their life. It is the point where many have reached the top of their career and/or become the head of the family, and are potentially caring for both older parents and children. This results in the younger person with dementia having a unique experience of dementia, as they try to understand and manage their symptoms with their role in society. This chapter will discuss the unique experience of younger people with dementia and their families, highlighting how this may be different from a person with later onset dementia. In particular, this will look at issues surrounding employment, finances, family life and getting a diagnosis, while highlighting the potential to live well with younger onset dementia with the appropriate care and support.

Getting a diagnosis

> I went to my GP because I was worried about my memory, she said it was due to work-related stress. It was only after I went back six months later with the same problems she referred me for tests.
>
> Younger person with dementia

For many people with younger onset dementia and their families the process of getting a diagnosis can be lengthy and challenging (Roach et al. 2014). While the process of diagnosis may be similar to those with later onset dementia, younger people more commonly have problems with misdiagnosis or trouble being referred to appropriate memory clinics. This is because many services are specifically for older adults (over 65) and adult services are not experienced in the diagnosis of dementia. Similarly, because early onset dementia is not as common, it is important that all other potential causes are ruled out before a diagnosis of dementia is made to a younger person. This means that when an individual experiences problems with cognition they are often mis-diagnosed (Mendez 2006). Often when an individual is treated for problems such as depression, work-related stress or anxiety the memory or cognitive problems prompting further investigation. For many females, symptoms of the menopause can emerge at the same time as they are experiencing initial symptoms of dementia that can further complicate diagnosis.

As a result of these challenges with diagnosis, many people with young onset dementia report the diagnostic process can take many months, and sometimes years. This, therefore presents challenges in other areas of their lives, where they are experiencing the symptoms of dementia but do not have an explanation for them.

Employment

> I'm not sure how long I can continue, but I love my job. It keeps my brain active and I think that helps.
>
> Josephine, 58, Office Manager

It is likely that a person diagnosed with dementia before the age of 65 will still be in employment. Therefore it is likely that they will require additional support with their employment, and similarly, their employer may need support as to how best to support their employee. Up until recently, much of what has been written about younger people with dementia has assumed that continuing employment is not possible following a diagnosis of dementia. This is because the majority of people with younger onset dementia do not continue working post diagnosis, for a variety of reasons. Individuals report feeling "pushed out" of employment after they receive a diagnosis (Bentham and La Fontaine 2006). Many other people have already left employment by the time they receive their diagnosis, either on sick leave or being made redundant, because they have been unable to cope with the stress of work alongside the unexplained symptoms they are experiencing (Ohman et al. 2003; Chaplin and Davidson 2014). A premature exit from the workforce will have many financial and social implications for the individual and their families which will be addressed later in this chapter.

Recent research has found that continued employment post diagnosis of dementia is possible with appropriate and timely support (Ritchie et al. 2017) (see Box 19.1 for more details). Supporting continued employment can be complex and involve employers having an understanding of dementia, a good relationship between the employee and employer, well planned adjustments and support from a wider network of collea-gues and the employee's family.

However, because of the complexities of dementia, and the range of employment an individual may be engaged in, it is difficult to make any generalisations about what an adjustment for an employee with dementia may be. This needs to be assessed on a person-centred basis, taking into account the job description, the individual's abilities and the support available within the workplace. Table 19.1 shows some examples of workplace adjustments that have been successful in supporting individuals with dementia to remain in employment.

Table 19.1 Examples of workplace adjustments in different workplaces

Job	Adjustment
Factory worker	Buddy system – employees are buddied with a colleague to provide support and check their tasks are completed.
Office workers	Flexible working – allowing the employee to work from home to avoid the commute to the office and to allow them to avoid the environmental distractions in the office.
Managerial jobs	Assistive technology – online calendars and diaries to provide memory prompts for work required and meetings.

Box 19.1 Research spotlight: Dementia in the workplace

Dementia in the Workplace was a research study that aimed to investigate the employment-related experiences of people with dementia post diagnosis with the view to understanding the potential for continued employment post diagnosis.

Seventeen case studies were conducted of people with dementia under the age of 65 who were still in employment or who had been in the previous 18 months. Interviews were carried out with the person with dementia, a family member and a representative from the workplace.

Of the 17 case studies, eight individuals continued employment post diagnosis while the other nine left employment either at the point of diagnosis or before. The key findings from across case analysis of the data are as follows:

1   While there were many similarities in situations, each case study revealed a different experience of employment post diagnosis of dementia.
2   Continued employment post diagnosis of dementia is possible, but can be complex to manage and dependent on a number of factors.
3   The participants who continued employment felt there were many benefits of continued employment. These included helping them to manage their symptoms, keeping connected, financial security and improved overall wellbeing.
4   For some participants, continued employment was not possible, and for others the stress of continuing employment had a negative effect on their wellbeing. In these cases, the participants felt poorly supported for leaving work and adjusting to retirement.
5   Employers and colleagues need support in order to support a person with dementia in the workplace. This support may include dementia awareness training, accessible information and practical guidance.

There are obvious financial benefits for continuing employment post diagnosis, which will be discussed later in this chapter. However, there are also potential social and psychological benefits to individuals who continue employment. The majority of participants who continued employment in the Ritchie et al. (2017) study reported that they felt continued employment helped them maintain their cognitive abilities, or control the symptoms of dementia. Others showed the benefit of increased social contact, helping them maintain their social networks and provide a feeling of normalcy to their lives. However, it should be noted that this is only based on the perceptions of the individuals with dementia, and there is no way of understanding the relationship between continued employment and these outcomes identified by the individuals.

At present, there is little known about the attitudes of employers towards supporting employees with dementia. Historically, dementia has not been considered a workplace issue, however with initiative such as Dementia Friends and Dementia-Friendly Communities in the UK, increasing numbers of businesses and employers are considering the impacts that dementia may have on their employees and business. Much of this work is focusing on how businesses can support customers with dementia, however a better understanding of dementia could also enable employers to support their employees affected by dementia as well. There is evidence to suggest that dementia awareness training is helpful for employers of individuals with dementia, in that it can help them better understand the challenges their employee is facing and support better decision making over reasonable adjustments to support their employee.

For a younger person with dementia, their employment situation post diagnosis can have a significant impact on their wider financial, family and social situation as well. As said previously, although it is possible for some people with dementia to continue working, poor support and understanding of the impact dementia has on an employee means that the current situation is that the majority of people with dementia do not continue employment post diagnosis. The following sections will examine the impact of a diagnosis of young onset dementia on family life, finances and social life.

Finances

> We used to have a comfortable lifestyle, now with the loss of my income we are struggling to make ends meet and make the mortgage payment each month.
>
> Younger person with dementia

If a diagnosis of young onset dementia results in loss of employment, this can result financial difficulties for the family. Many younger people with dementia take early retirement following diagnosis. While this may be the best option for many people, it will result in a reduction in income over the lifetime. Families may still have outstanding mortgages, and the loss of income may make it difficult to keep up with mortgage payments and other outgoings. As household income is restricted this will have a wider impact on the lifestyle and quality of life of the family or individual. Extreme circumstances could result in loss of the family home.

If an individual loses employment, and is not eligible for early-retirement or does not have an adequate pension, they will have to then negotiate the benefits system to maintain their income. Younger people with dementia have reported difficulties in accessing appropriate advice and support with regard to benefits and have often felt stigmatised, where assessors do not understand their disability or they are subjected to stressful assessments that expect them to rely on their memory to complete.

Family life

> I am now the only income for the family. It's difficult juggling work, caring for the family and supporting my husband with dementia. I'm not sure how long I will manage to keep it all going.
>
> Wife of younger person with dementia

For all families, someone being diagnosed with dementia can change their way of life and affect relationships and lifestyle. This is the same when a member of the family is diagnosed with young onset dementia. However, a younger person with dementia is likely to have a different family dynamic and lifestyle from a person who is diagnosed in their seventies or eighties. A younger person with dementia may still have dependent children, their spouse or partner is more likely to still be in employment and the family may have a number of outstanding financial commitments.

Spouses and partners of younger people with dementia report increased stress levels as they attempt to support their spouse. There are a number of issues to consider here. Firstly, the impact this may have on their own employment. The transition to becoming a carer of a younger person with dementia will mean that they may need to request flexible working to support their partner going to appointments, or provide assistance with tasks, such as supporting them to get ready in the morning, or ensuring they remember to eat their lunch.

Spouses of individuals with younger onset dementia face many of the same problems as those caring for an individual with later onset dementia, such as, getting a diagnosis, adapting to the care giving role, and adjusting to changes in their partners behaviour. Research has shown that the impact of these problems is potentially more disruptive and severe for those caring for someone with early onset dementia (Roach et al. 2014). In particular, younger caregiver age is associated with higher incidence of depression, and an increased sense of stigma surrounding the diagnosis, both in how they adapt to the caregiver role and how they perceive their spouse being treated in society. Spouses also report increased worry about the stability of their employment and how long they will be able to continue working as their partner's dementia progresses. Partners of younger people with dementia often report giving up activities such as employment or other social activities to either avoid leaving their spouse at home, or changing arrangements or activities to ensure they are able to include their spouse (Hawkins 2012).

Many people in society are now choosing to have children later in life, in their late thirties and forties. If an individual is diagnosed with dementia in their fifties, this means that there is a chance they could still have children who are in school or further education who are reliant on them financially and emotionally. There is very little known about the experiences of children or young adults who have a parent with young onset dementia. However, a recent study has attempted to address this gap (Box 19.2).

Box 19.2 Research spotlight: Children of younger people with dementia – Perceptions and experiences of children and young people with a parent with dementia

The aim of this study was to understand the perceptions and experiences of children and young people who have a parent with dementia.

Nineteen interviews were held with individuals who had a parent with dementia. Participants were aged between eight and 31 and interviews took an autobiographical approach to collect in-depth narratives on the experiences of the participants.

A thematic analysis of the data identified the following eight themes:

1   Not the same person – participants had difficulty in accepting the narrative that their parent was "still the same person".
2   They had to "Hollywood" it – in reference to the recent media attention on young onset dementia through the film *Still Alice*.
3   My parent is a different person – participants expressed grief at the changing role of their parent in their life.
4   My parent doesn't know me – participants spoke of grief or fear at the thought that their parent will no longer recognise them as their child.

The final four themes related to problems the participants identified with dealing with the impacts of their parents' symptoms on their relationship.

5   My parent isn't very nice.
6   My parent is aggressive.
7   My parent is suspicious.
8   My parent can't talk to me.

(Sikes & Hall 2018)

Children and young adults with a parent with young onset dementia experience a range of emotions, including grief at the change in the child-parent relationship. This includes sadness at their parent's lack of ability to support them through milestones in their life, including graduations, marriage, birth of grandchildren etc. Additionally, they may experience anger or embarrassment at their parent's behaviour. In essence, young onset dementia can change the parent-child relationship dynamic where the child perceives the parent as 'changed' and unable to provide the support they require (Sikes & Hall 2018).

Providing support for the family, including children is important post diagnosis of young onset dementia. Children can experience increased stress and fear when their parent is diagnosed, as well as increased concern for the wellbeing of their parent who does not have dementia (Allen et al 2009). Additionally, children have reported feeling neglected in the process of diagnosis and post diagnostic support, feeling ill-informed and helpless (Barca et al. 2014). However, this could be alleviated by adopting a whole family approach to post diagnostic support, which incorporates dementia services and family and children's services. By doing so, children can receive age appropriate information about their parent's diagnosis and the likely progression of the disease. It is also suggested that providing peer support groups for children who have a parent with dementia is a useful support strategy.

So far this section has focused on the impact of a diagnosis of young onset dementia within a family unit. However, increasing numbers of people in mid-life are living alone, and therefore many younger people with dementia may live alone. This group of people are often overlooked in research as they are often more difficult to access as participants and therefore little is known about their experiences of living alone. For these younger people living alone, there is an increased chance of social isolation and care must be taken to ensure they are well supported in the community.

Social life and activity

> All my friends are still working, so I don't get the chance to see them very often. I need to find other things to fill the days now.
>
> Younger person with dementia

The younger person with dementia and their families may find their social lives altered. This is in terms of social networks, and the availability of age-appropriate activities. One of the major issues in the care of people with younger onset dementia is the lack of age-appropriate services following diagnosis. In many areas, diagnosis of dementia comes through older person's healthcare services, regardless of age. This means a person who is 55 could be referred to a clinic that is designed for people who may be a generation older than him or her. This pattern is often echoed in dementia services in the community. Many younger people with dementia are, understandably, reluctant to attend dementia cafes, and other support or activity groups that are designed for and attended by much older people. This can result in increased social isolation for the individual with dementia, where no alternative is identified. This may be more pronounced in males, who are more likely to have their social life interlinked with their work life and loss of employment can also result in loss of their social networks (Ritchie et al. 2017).

People with dementia and their families frequently report a loss of social contact post diagnosis, where well-meaning friends attempt to keep contact but this gradually reduces until there is very little contact between friends (Hawkins 2012). The loss of employment and loss of other social activities can result in negative consequences for individuals with young onset dementia, including increased instances of depression and feelings of loss of power and identity. For many people, these losses are reported as more significant than the financial losses of employment (Greenwood and Smith 2016). However, although many younger people with dementia go through a period of loss and grieving post diagnosis, the emerging research and policy in the area is increasingly highlighting the living the best life possible message. The importance of peer support groups for younger people with dementia and their families is increasingly being highlighted and much research focuses on creating a new normal and focusing on new interests and creating new social connections (Pipon-Young et al. 2012; Roach & Drummond 2014). Finding activities which are meaningful for younger people with dementia needs to take into account the stage of life they are at, previous experiences and interests and availability of services.

Box 19.3 Social media and younger people with dementia

In recent years, the increase in the use of social media has helped many younger people with dementia to get their voice heard in a public forum and has helped to promote the "Living Well with Dementia" message as well as using it to influence public attitudes towards dementia and policy and research priorities. Examples of blogs written by younger people with dementia are:

Kate Swaffer, "Creating Life with Words: Inspiration, Love and Truth." Available from: https://kateswaffer.com/daily-blog/.
Wendy Mitchell: "Which me am I today?." Available from: https://whichmeamitoday.wordpress.com/.

As society becomes more technological focused, many people with early onset dementia find they are using everyday technology and social media to create social networks, interact and raise awareness of their life with young onset dementia. People such as Kate Swaffer and Wendy Mitchell (see Box 19.3) are regular bloggers and have a large social media following. Because younger people with dementia are more likely to be physically fit and more familiar with technology, younger people with dementia are more able to be visible in this way. Therefore, the voices of people with young onset dementia are more frequently being heard through the media and are influencing dementia policy on a national and international basis. Being able to provide an insight to living with younger onset dementia has a role to play in addressing the stigma of dementia and promoting a dementia-aware community.

Conclusion

This chapter has attempted to provide an insight into the lives of people living with younger onset dementia. While it has attempted to touch on the broad issues which make a diagnosis of young onset dementia a unique experience to people diagnosed in later life, it is important to remember that everyone who receives a diagnosis will have their own unique experience. A diagnosis of younger onset dementia is a life-changing event, however here we have described that with the correct care and support, living well with younger onset dementia is possible.

References

Allen, J., Oyebode, J.R. and Allen, J. (2009) "Having a father with young onset dementia: the impact on well-being of young people." *Dementia*, 8(4): 455–480. doi.org/10.1177/1471301209349106

Barca, M.L., Thorsen, K., Engedal, K., Haugen, P.K. and Johannessen, A. (2014) "Nobody asked me how I felt: experiences of adult children of persons with young-onset dementia." *International psychogeriatrics*, 26(12): 1935–1944.

Bentham, P. and La Fontaine, J. (2007) "Service development for younger people with dementia." *Psychiatry*, 7(2): 84–87.

Cabote, C. J., Bramble, M. and McCann, D. (2015) "Family caregivers' experiences of caring for a relative with younger onset dementia." *Journal of Family Nursing*, 21(3): 443–468.

Chaplin, R. and Davidson, I. (2014) "What are the experiences of people with dementia in employment?" *Dementia*, 15(2): 147–161. doi:10.1177/1471301213519252.

Ducharme, F., Kergoat, M.-J., Antoine, P., Pasquier, F. and Coulombe, R. (2013) "The unique experience of spouses in early-onset dementia." *American Journal of Alzheimer's Disease and Other Dementias*, 28(6): 634–641.

Erikson, E.H., Paul, I.H., Heider, F., and Gardner, R.W. (1959) *Psychological Issues* (Vol. 1). New York: International Universities Press.

Greenwood, N. and Smith, R. (2016) "The experiences of people with young-onset dementia: A meta-ethnographic review of the qualitative literature." *Maturitas*, 92, 102–109.

Harris, P. B. and Keady, J. (2009) "Selfhood in younger onset dementia: transitions and testimonies." *Aging and Mental Health*, 13(3): 437–444.

Hawkins, S.A., (2012) "The social experiences of spouses of persons with young-onset dementia." (PhD thesis).

Mendez, M.F. (2006) "The accurate diagnosis of early-onset dementia." *The International Journal of Psychiatry in Medicine*, 36(4): 401–412.

Millenaar, J.K., van Vliet, D., Bakker, C., Vernooij-Dassen, M.J., Koopmans, R.T., Verhey, F.R. and de Vugt, M.E. (2014) "The experiences and needs of children living with a parent with young onset dementia: results from the NeedYD study." *International Psychogeriatrics*, 26(12): 2001–2010.

Ohman, A., Nygard, L. and Borell, L. (2003) "The vocational situation in cases of memory deficits or younger-onset dementia." *Scandinavian Journal of Caring Sciences*, 15(1): 34–43.

Pipon-Young, F. E., Lee, K. M., Jones, F. and Guss, R. (2012) "I'm not all gone, I can still speak: The experiences of younger people with Dementia. An action research study." *Dementia*, 11(5): 597–616.

Ritchie, L., Tolson, D., and Danson, M. (2017) "Dementia in the workplace case study research: understanding the experiences of individuals, colleagues and managers." *Ageing and Society*, 1(30). doi:10.1017/S0144686X17000563.

Roach, P. and Drummond, N. (2014) "'It's nice to have something to do': early-onset dementia and maintaining purposeful activity." *Journal of Psychiatric and Mental Health Nursing*, 21(10): 889–895.

Roach, P., Keady, J., Bee, P. and Williams, S. (2014) "'We can't keep going on like this': identifying family storylines in young onset dementia." *Ageing and Society*, 34(08): 1397–1426.

Sikes, P. and Hall, M. (2018) "'It was then that I thought "whaat? This is not my Dad"': The implications of the 'still the same person' narrative for children and young people who have a parent with dementia." *Dementia*, 17(2): 180–198.

Further reading

Hayo, H., Ward, A. and Parkes, J. (2018) *Young Onset Dementia*. London: Jessica Kingsley Publishers.

Mitchell, W. (2018) *Somebody that I used to know*. Bloomsbury: London.

Young Dementia UK. Available from: https://www.youngdementiauk.org/.

20 Down's syndrome and dementia

Karen Watchman and Sam Quinn

Introduction

People with Down's syndrome are enjoying a longer life expectancy than ever before, with many living beyond 60 years, a marked change from life expectancy of just 25 in 1983. Along with greater longevity comes awareness that a disproportionately high number of individuals with Down's syndrome will have dementia by their mid-fifties. This challenges not only the individual affected, but also health and social care service providers and families who are required to change their caring role, often with limited additional support if the family has previously been considered to cope well.

Many of the current older population of people with Down's syndrome will not have had a baseline assessment in their thirties, as is now recommended. In this chapter we focus on the fictitious case study of Robbie, a 46-year-old man with Down's syndrome and dementia living alone with outreach support from a social care provider and with family nearby. Robbie did not have a baseline assessment before he started to experience changes; we consider the critical issues that need to be addressed by Robbie, by his service provider, peers and family. This includes discussion of how far Robbie can consider his accommodation a "home for life", and the changes required to enable this: environmentally through design adaptations, socially by staff supporting Robbie and his peers, and emotionally by Robbie and his family.

In considering these issues, it is highlighted how people with Down's syndrome, and other learning disabilities, may experience dementia differently to people who do not have any learning disability. This includes differences in: age of onset, pre- and co-existing health conditions, living arrangements, understanding of dementia, role of family and previous experience of inclusion in healthcare decisions.

Current knowledge

Down's syndrome is a condition that is present from birth and is caused by the presence of all or part of an extra copy of chromosome 21. Average life expectancy has increased due to screening that is now routine at birth with medical intervention as required, for example for congenital heart defects. Life expectancy is also extended due to enhanced quality of life and positive experiences brought about as a result of advocacy and self-advocacy that far outweigh previous lifestyles of institutional living and lack of opportunity.

Along with this awareness comes knowledge of a range of age-related health issues that typically affect some people with Down's syndrome more frequently than other types of learning disability. One notable issue is the increased potential to develop dementia at an earlier age. Around one third of people with Down's syndrome aged between 55 and 59 have a diagnosis of dementia. Although the reason for this is not well understood, it is related to chromosome 21. The extra DNA on chromosome 21 leads to an overdevelopment of the protein amyloid precursor protein, which forms plaques on the brain.

Whilst we do not fully understand the function of amyloid precursor protein, we know that day-to-day brain activity involves a continual processing of amyloid precursor protein into shorter pieces. In doing so, one of the processing pathways produces beta-amyloid, which is responsible for Alzheimer-related changes. As a result, individuals with Down's syndrome who have an extra copy of the amyloid precursor protein gene may have increased production of beta-amyloid, resulting in a higher likelihood of developing Alzheimer's disease. We also know that the frontal lobes of people with Down's syndrome are smaller and under-developed in relation to individuals of the same age without Down's syndrome, something that is exacerbated with ageing. This may explain personality or behavioural changes that can occur for people with Down's syndrome and dementia, for example increased irritability.

Introducing Robbie

Robbie is a 46-year-old man with Down's syndrome. He grew up in his family home with both parents and two older siblings. He had always planned to move out and live independently "like my brothers". This became a reality at age 32 when he moved to his own flat eight miles from his parents, with daily outreach support from a third sector learning disability service provider.

His Community Learning Disability Nurse and social care staff became concerned that he was not cleaning his flat. He often appeared dishevelled and was late for college. He started having difficulty remembering the days of the week or what he had eaten earlier that day and became prone to aggressive outbursts which were considered to be out of character. He was also talking aloud more to himself. At home, Robbie became increasingly nervous moving around his flat and needed to hold on to furniture in order to move around the room. His balance was affected and he started experiencing dizzy spells.

Box 20.1 Perspective of Robbie's family

Robbie's parents aged 84 and 87 were initially reluctant to seek any help to understand these changes; they were not aware of the higher risk of dementia in people with Down's syndrome. They had not expected Robbie to outlive them having been told when he was born that he "would be lucky to reach adulthood". They acknowledge that he has been over-protected to the extent that they now understood the changes they had been observing, and compensating for, over a two-year period were likely to be dementia-related. However, his brothers, one of whom was Robbie's welfare guardian, knew of the link and were persistent in the need to seek help.

Changing health

There is a need to differentiate between changes that are due to ageing generally and changes that may be attributed to a type of dementia. A baseline assessment is recommended that records typical functioning and behaviour when in good health, followed by a review every two years, up to age 50 for people with Down's syndrome, then annually thereafter to monitor any changes to the baseline that may indicate dementia. Equally important are regular reviews that may identify a treatable condition that may have otherwise been missed, such as changes to vision, onset of diabetes or change in thyroid functioning.

Robbie did not have a baseline assessment when he was younger as this has only been a recent adoption in his health board locality. Standard tests of cognitive ability that could have indicated dementia were not appropriate due to Robbie's learning disability, as he would not have been able to take the tests even before dementia was suspected. Therefore a different approach was required. This involved eliminating, or treating, other conditions that may mimic dementia. This can be a time consuming process and, if dementia is also present may delay a diagnosis by months or even years.

Eyesight and hearing were checked first of all – Robbie did not have the correct glasses prescription and was found to have an ear infection; associated dizziness was affecting his balance. People with Down's syndrome have smaller ear canals so hearing should be routinely checked. Other conditions, commonly seen in people with Down's syndrome that were ruled out included keratoconus (coning of the cornea resulting in a "bulging" eye) and cataracts (when the lens of the eye changes, resulting in blurry or misty vision).

Although Robbie was overweight and could occasionally become constipated, he did not have major gastrointestinal disorders such as coeliac disease, inflammatory bowel disease or reflux, all of which people with Down's syndrome are susceptible to. Self-talk, or speaking aloud to no one in particular, is not uncommon in people with Down's syndrome and typically, unless a drastic change in tone or frequency, is adaptive rather a cause for concern and often viewed as a coping mechanism. As this behaviour was not new for Robbie, it was not associated with the onset of dementia.

Box 20.2 Good practice checklist

- There needs to be a distinction between what could be the onset of dementia and other health or sensory conditions that Robbie may be experiencing. Without this, treatment cannot be tailored to his specific condition(s) and a diagnosis of dementia may overshadow other treatable health conditions.
- Support for Robbie and his family during the diagnosis phase is crucial with explanations needed in the most accessible way to aid understanding of changes that are experienced.
- Pharmacological interventions should be discussed with Robbie's GP following assessment and only after ruling out, or identifying, health or sensory conditions and should be regularly reviewed.
- Non-pharmacological supports should be discussed with Robbie's Community Learning Disability Nurse and Allied Health professionals.

- Planning for the future should have Robbie at the centre; this includes consideration of what is needed to enable him to exercise personal choice and have input into any decisions made using individualised methods of communication.

This tool, the Early Detection Screen for Dementia was developed by the National Task Group as a screening instrument suitable for use by family or staff to identify early signs and symptoms of dementia in adults with intellectual disabilities. It can be used to help identify those individuals with dementia-like symptoms whose function and behaviour are the results of other causes such as thyroid disorders, medication interactions, depression and other co-existing conditions. In Robbie's case, the version adapted for use in Scotland (Watchman et al. 2018) alerted his siblings to changes associated with his thyroid, eyesight and his ear infection that led to a dialogue with health care practitioners and helped to identify changes that were, and were not, associated with the onset of dementia.

Post-diagnostic pharmacological interventions

After a process of assessment from a learning disability psychiatrist, and drawing on evidence and experience of Robbie, his families and his support network, a probable diagnosis of dementia was made and medication was discussed with his family. Much of the research and clinical trials on medication for dementia has been with people who do not have a learning disability.

Since May 2016, Donepezil, Galantamine and Rivastigmine have been recommended in the UK as options for managing mild as well as moderate Alzheimer's disease, and Memantine is now recommended as an option for managing moderate Alzheimer's disease for patients who are unable to take AChE inhibitors, and as an option for managing severe Alzheimer's disease. However, a trial of Memantine that including people with dementia and Down's syndrome and dementia did not report any benefit. Although there is not a strong clinical evidence base, and the evidence that exists is largely with people who have Down's syndrome rather than other types of learning disability, anecdotal evidence suggests that there may be some positive outcomes to prescribing Donepezil (also known as Aricept) although side effects can be extreme and must be monitored closely.

This was the course of action followed with Robbie who was prescribed Aricept with his parents, brothers and support staff alerted to possible side effects that include abdominal pain, diarrhoea, aggression or urinary incontinence. For the first four weeks Robbie experienced dizzy spells, loss of appetite and increased restlessness at night. When reviewed, it was agreed to continue as Robbie was able to tolerate the former two side effects.

Post-diagnostic non-pharmacological supports

As with people who have dementia but not a learning disability, social support and companionship remain important, but appropriate activities may not be immediately obvious. Although the guiding principles remain the same for non-pharmacological interventions, there may be differences in implementation with people who have both a learning disability and dementia.

General principles for supporting a person with dementia include looking at the environment, both in terms of signage and colour contrast for wayfinding, and also a quiet calm setting. Although people with dementia can experience sensory overload in situations that others experience as low background noise it is equally important that stimulation is appropriate for the individual – what is right for one person will be too noisy / quiet for another.

Robbie's support staff were already aware of the need for a calm environment and had transferred some of their learning from supporting a resident with autism to supporting Robbie with dementia. This included adapting social communication, understanding the risk of over or under-sensitivity to sound, touch, taste smell, light or colour, the importance of a fixed routine and repeated activity. What they did not recognise was that this would need to be reviewed on a much more regular basis and that long-term strategies that had been in place for many years would need to change as dementia progressed. This meant that support, although individualised in terms of Robbie's preferred music and his love of animals was continuing as it had done for many years rather than adapting as his needs changed. Consequently, he became increasingly irritable and showed agitation when music was played for too long, even though it was his favourite singer or when the visiting pet therapy dog paid attention to anyone else.

Box 20.3 Good practice checklist

- The guiding principles for environmental design to support people with dementia are the same whether the individual has a learning disability or not – where the person with dementia lives or spends time should be: calm, familiar, predictable and appropriately stimulating.
- However, although creating a quiet, calm environment is important this should not be to the extent that there is no stimulation at all for the person – the balance is ensuring appropriate stimulation for the individual. What is right for one person will be too noisy or confusing for another.
- Activities and interventions should be reviewed – individual needs and preferences can change with the progression of dementia.
- Support staff should build on their existing skills and experiences and not necessarily start again with strategies or interventions.
- Brighter lighting and maximising natural light can counteract loss of visual acuity with age, but may also increase confidence in movement and mobility if the surrounding area is more visible.
- Resource centres or daytime/volunteering/employment activities can become difficult due to noise and activity levels, but if the person affected by dementia is able to remain focused on an enjoyable activity that is meaningful to them without necessarily the requirement to move around, attendance may be facilitated for longer.

Supporting Robbie to have a voice

Robbie lives alone, a number of his friends who also have a learning disability live in adjoining flats. They meet as a group regularly at both planned events and informally as neighbours, often providing informal support for each other. As Robbie's health has changed he has become more withdrawn and less interested in social activities. Robbie was aware that "something is wrong" although his family were always quick to reassure him that he was fine; they did not want to worry him and were unsure of how to broach the issue of dementia. It was important to understand the best way of ensuring that Robbie's wishes and preferences were heard and that he understood why he was experiencing changes even if he did not understand the word *dementia*.

Robbie's Community Learning Disability Nurse gave his family a copy of *Jenny's Diary*, a pictorial resource to support conversations about dementia with people who have a learning disability. Figure 20.1 shows the model that can be followed and adapted by Robbie's family to explain the diagnosis of dementia to Robbie and his friends. This involves using Robbie's existing knowledge to agree an approach that would explain to Robbie that he was ill, and explain to his friends why Robbie was less outgoing and more irritable than usual.

In the early stages of dementia, support from peers can be productive and can facilitate the person with a learning disability affected by dementia to maintain social contacts and activities. However, this should be monitored as the opposite may occur as dementia progresses; being in a busy environment or in the company of too many people may have a detrimental effect on Robbie's wellbeing. This will also require a different explanation given to peers as dementia advances to acknowledge associated changes in Robbie's behaviour towards them.

Box 20.4 Good practice checklist

- Feeling uncomfortable or nervous about talking with a person who has a learning disability about dementia is understandable, however, such conversations can help the individual or friend come to terms with a diagnosis.
- Be consistent in the terms or words used to talk to Robbie; friends, support staff and family should use the same words.
- Support friends or a partner with a learning disability in their own right, their concerns and needs will be different to those experienced by Robbie.
- Depending on the understanding of the person with a learning disability, it may, or may not, be appropriate to use the word "dementia" in an explanation of the health changes being experienced.
- Often the most important thing is to help make sense of the changes that are being experienced on that day.
- Keep asking the question, whether among family, friends or professionals "what can we do to help Robbie feel safe, less confused and less frightened?"

Home for good?

Robbie has lived in his current home for 14 years and wants to stay there, to "age in place". Ageing in place is an approach that aims to help a person stay in their accommodation for as long as possible with appropriate support provided as their needs progress. However, he has an upstairs bedroom and is already having difficulty with the stairs. He uses the lift but has become fearful of it recently.

This approach requires increasingly specialised support for changing health and social care needs. Up until now Robbie has been helped to maintain the tenancy of his flat with the assistance of family and social care staff, however, his brothers have raised

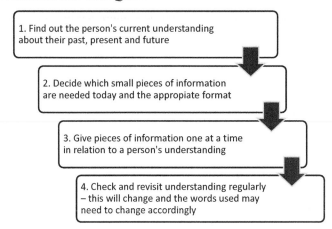

1. Find out the person's current understanding about their past, present and future

2. Decide which small pieces of information are needed today and the appropiate format

3. Give pieces of information one at a time in relation to a person's understanding

4. Check and revisit understanding regularly – this will change and the words used may need to change accordingly

Figure 20.1 A stepped model for sharing information about the diagnosis of dementia with people who have a learning disability
Source: Watchman et al. (2015).

concern about the suitability of the flat due to the number of stairs and the lack of 24-hour support, particularly overnight. A case conference called by his Community Learning Disability Nurse identified areas where additional support could be provided.

This included environmental adaptations such as improved lighting in his dark hallway, an increase in the size of signage, a telephone with photographs rather than numbers to enable him to call family or staff quickly if needed. Mirrored walls were covered in the lift to minimise confusion, the lift door sensor was changed to enable more time for the person entering and leaving, and a small seat was added for comfort. After discussion with other tenants in the building Robbie was encouraged to add some pictures and posters to the lift interior – he chose to add images of his favourite football team. His photograph was added alongside the button to be pressed to reach his floor.

Currently this is facilitating Robbie's ongoing use of the lift, he is no longer afraid of the darkness, the confusing effect of the mirrors, the number of buttons or the doors that closed too quickly, instead he sees a bright, comfortable and familiar space that makes sense to him. However, his family realise that this may not be a long-term option. With no downstairs rooms available Robbie's brothers are aware that this accommodation, although Robbie's long-term home and his preferred place to be, may not always be the most appropriate space in the future. When looking at where people with a learning disability and dementia live two other models of care are prominent in addition to ageing in place: referral out and in place progression.

Referral out means that a person with a learning disability and dementia is moved to a care home. While this option typically sees higher resident turnover meaning shorter waiting lists for new residents especially in emergency situations, it also typically means a person with Down's syndrome (for example) living in a care home with other residents who are in their eighties and nineties. Robbie's brothers have concerns about this as a viable option due to the significant age difference between Robbie and other residents and their uncertainty over whether staff in an aged care facility are suitably trained and confident at supporting a resident with Down's syndrome.

In place progression is an approach based around a group of individuals, ideally with a similar level of need, sharing a dementia-specific environment. This model is increasingly being seen or considered among service providers in the UK as a means of ensuring that the individual remains there until end of life rather than moving elsewhere, often in a crisis situation. Whilst Robbie's care providers were discussing developing a dementia-specific service due to the increasing number of older people they were supporting with a learning disability and dementia, this was not yet available to the family.

Box 20.5 Reflective questions

- To continue to facilitate feeling safe at home in the longer term may require environmental changes or even a move elsewhere; how can we start this process of thinking ahead to longer term health, social care and accommodation needs thus avoiding crisis situations later?
- We have seen that families and staff should be supported to adapt or find suitable accommodation as dementia progresses in the person with a learning disability they care for. How can we make appropriate physical adaptions to an existing environment introduce the possibility of alternate accommodation that may be more suited to the individual's needs?

Summary

By using the example of Robbie, and highlighting his changing needs, we have identified similarities and differences between people with and without Down's syndrome affected by dementia. Differences includes earlier onset, the potential overshadowing of co-existing health conditions, differences in the way in which dementia is diagnosed and the role of a baseline in the diagnostic process under-standing of dementia and for some, already different or adapted communication methods.

Increasingly people with Down's syndrome will have a baseline as a young adult from which to measure changes in health; this is in place of the standard cognitive functioning tests taken by people without a learning disability. However, we have seen from Robbie's example that not having a baseline assessment when younger is not a barrier to making a diagnosis or putting support in place in the short, medium and longer term.

Indeed, over time so may the individual's understanding of what is happening to them change. As in Robbie's case, a diagnosis of dementia can also affect friends and peers. Utilising an appropriate framework and giving information about the diagnosis to the person with Down's syndrome, even if this is as needed on a day-to-day basis, respects the right of all people to know of their diagnosis in a way that is appropriate and supportive.

We have considered the critical issues that Robbie, his family, peers and service provider should address in order to help Robbie live well with dementia now and in the future. Through careful monitoring of his medication, non-pharmacological support and appropriate environmental adaptions, an individual with Down's syndrome and dementia may continue to age in place in a familiar and comfortable environment and have a "home for life". Where support is already in place, due to the existing learning disability, there needs to be recognition that it cannot continue at the same level and changes will be needed as dementia progresses.

References

Watchman, K., Tuffrey-Wijne, I. and Quinn, S. (2015) *Jenny's diary: Supporting conversations about dementia with people who have a learning disability.* London: Alzheimer's Society. Available from: http://www.uws.ac.uk/jennysdiary/.

Watchman, K., Ewing, J., and Scotland, S. (2018) "The NTG-Early Detection Screen for Dementia – Scottish version adapted from National Task Group on Intellectual Disabilities and Dementia Practices (2012) NTG -EDSD Screening Instrument." Available from: http://aadmd.org/sites/default/files/NTG-EDSD-Final-Scotland%202018.pdf.

Further reading

Alzheimer's Society. (2015) "Intellectual disability and dementia factsheet." Available from: https://www.alzheimers.org.uk/info/20007/types_of_dementia/37/learning_disabilities_and_dementia.

Foundation for People with Learning Disabilities. (2013) "Thinking ahead: supporting families to plan for the future." Available from: https://www.mentalhealth.org.uk/learning-disabilities/our-work/family-friends-community/thinking-ahead/.

Watchman, K. (2017) *Intellectual Disability and Dementia: A Guide for Families.* London: Jessica Kingsley Publishers.

Watchman, K., Kerr, D. and Wilkinson, H. (2010) *Supporting Derek.* University of Edinburgh: Joseph Rowntree Foundation.

Watchman, K., Tuffrey-Wijne, I. and Quinn, S. (2015) *Jenny's diary: Supporting conversations about dementia with people who have a learning disability.* London: Alzheimer's Society. Available from: http://www.uws.ac.uk/jennysdiary/.

21 Dementia and human rights

The view from someone who is living with dementia

James McKillop

This chapter has been largely written by someone who has dementia. James was a founding member of the Scottish Dementia Working Group, a campaigning group of people with dementia that is supported by Alzheimer Scotland. It describes the views of the group, as well as describing some of the issues faced by people with dementia.

Much is made of people *gaining* their human rights nowadays. But what about *losing* the human rights you enjoyed, before a certain, life-changing event happened? That is, a diagnosis of dementia.

A survey showed, it is the most feared illness, replacing cancer, which may be treatable. No wonder, when you see how people with dementia were treated in the past, and still are today. It is a deteriorating illness that may advance slowly or quickly. No one can predict which it will be. It is in the laps of the Gods.

Going back to 1906, a German doctor diagnosed the nature of the illness that would bear his name throughout the world – Dr Alois Alzheimer. Since then there have been great strides in both diagnosing and treating illnesses. Research concentrated on more fashionable diseases, but dementia was the Cinderella. Very little was done for many years, and it was round about 2000 that it began to be taken seriously.

Over the years health care has improved and people are living longer. But that is the biggest risk, inter alia, for developing dementia. The tsunami of cases around the world has led to research all over the globe. Every researcher is scrambling for a prevention and/or a cure. Prevention is better. Genetic research may come up with an answer, but there is currently no end in sight. We need another Dr Alexander Fleming.

So, until that magic day, we have to proceed with what we have now, and that is a timely diagnosis. What can happen? Your employer may want shod of you.

If you are self-employed, orders for work are down.

Friends may pretend not to see you in the street and pass by.

They may stop visiting.

Invitations to visits dry up.

They are uneasy if you drop in, and don't ask you to come back some day.

Invites to family gatherings, baptisms, marriage, funerals, birthday and anniversaries are "lost" in the post, as they fear what you might do or say, and act inappropriately.

You lose control of the household finances.

Your credit/debit card is cut up.

Your partner and any children, no longer seek your counsel.

Your immediate family might hide your car keys and maybe sell your car, or disable it.

Your grandchildren may find their marriage prospects in jeopardy ("it" may run in the family).

You may end up at the bottom of a waiting list for medical treatment/operations; others who are judged of more value to the community have priority.

In the mid twentieth century, cancer was the elephant in the room. The person with the illness was the last to know, if they were ever told at all. They were fobbed off with a euphemism like "a bit of a chest infection".

Dementia segued into the new elephant. Again, you weren't told the exact nature of the illness, just that you had a wee memory problem. You found your liberties were surreptitiously disappearing. Your day-to-day activities were being arranged by someone else. You had to tell them where you were going out to, and when you would return. Or someone suddenly accompanied you. You were reminded to take enough change for a small purchase such as a paper, and prevented from carrying too much money on you. Someone checked you had your hat on, a coat around your shoulders, gloves on your hands and to take an umbrella on bad days. Loose clothing, liquid and sun block on sunny days. People stopped being car passengers, and maybe you were asked to stop driving by your family. Children stopped you taking their children out with you in the car. And so on. Your role as a doting grandparent became liable to scrutiny at every step.

This is demoralising and you begin to feel a failure. You are letting people down and the rosy picture you dreamed of in retirement has faded.

But dementia is not the end of your life, it the start of a new life and will be what you make of it.

You can sit at home and mope, "why me?" and life will go downhill.

Or you can face up to the diagnosis, and get on with the rest of your life. It will not be an easy path and the illness is deteriorating. But you can look around you and see what is out there to help you cope. There will be regrets, but they should not dominate you. Concentrate on what skills you already have and be prepared to try something new, maybe something you have always wanted to experience, but never had the time. NOW IS THE TIME!

What is available in your area, what type of support would you like to have, to maintain as normal a life as possible? What do you want? No one can read your mind, you must be vocal.

Now in Scotland, you have a guaranteed right to a year's post diagnostic support from a trained Link Worker. Their raison d'être is to have an intimate knowledge of what is available in your area, to help you maintain your quality of life. You will have downs, but so do most happy people, it is the nature of the beast. But you will have highs you never ever dreamed of. Many people with dementia are doing things, such as public speaking, something they had never envisaged in their lives. Dementia can give you a new kind of courage.

What else do people with dementia want? In a few words, human rights. Not more than any citizen and certainly not less. Just our basic human rights. People with dementia can be regarded as non-productive, so when it comes to things like health care and operations, priority may be given to contributors to society.

If your home becomes unsuitable, you can be offered sub-standard accommodation. If you are in a group, you might be able to approach housing planners with models for the future in mind.

If you need to rely on benefits, the fact that we can walk and talk and look well, could count against a fair assessment of your needs. You might want to consider an advocate to assist you.

If you think you need some form of social care, consult your social work office. Do not be put off by the fact that it used to be a stigma having one. They are dedicated people, working to help all areas of the community.

If you want to fit in with your neighbours, they need to understand what dementia is and how it affects people and their well-being and behaviour. Dementia training should start at school primary level, aimed of course at their level, so that one day everyone in Scotland will have some basic knowledge of dementia. And more importantly, while the older generation may not have the knowledge unless it affects them personally, the new generations will know for eternity until, I pray, there is a prevention and/or a cure.

Finally, general health. While dementia can affect people in their thirties, forties and fifties although rarely so, age is the biggest risk factor. But old age does not come alone. There are all sorts of co-morbidities lying in wait, for everybody. The current thinking is to integrate health and social care, and this may be slow to happen in your area. So be abreast of the latest news.

Who decides what you are entitled to, to live your life? Initial decisions come from politicians. So, if something is affecting a lot of people, band together and let them know. They cannot lift a finger unless it is brought to their attention.

Part IV
Future practice

22 Advances in knowledge

Debbie Tolson and Graham A. Jackson

Introduction

The fact that worldwide over 46 million people are currently affected by dementia and that this number will rise to 75 million by 2030, makes dementia one of the biggest global public health challenges of the 21st century. It follows that advancing biomedical research that will inform prevention and cure dementia are central to the quest for new knowledge.

However, for people living with dementia today and those soon to be diagnosed, it is the generation of new applied knowledge from practice-based research that will influence their care experience and outcomes. Indeed, the immediacy of impact from practice based research, with its potential to influence policy, practice and experiences of care is pivotal to advancing health and social care and propelling integrated care. As you will appreciate from earlier chapters which promote rights-based approaches and foreground person-centred care delivered within a relational framework, we believe that an explicit value orientation should underpin both the generation of applied knowledge and its application within practice. The evidence used to inform practice is socially negotiated and aligns with current views on what constitutes knowledge (Nutley et al. 2003).

The nature of applied knowledge

Philosophers have long debated the nature of knowledge and ways of knowing and thinking about scientific truths. Some would argue that scientists, like all of us learn from their mistakes. A view that would perhaps worry patients if that was how treatment and care options were presented. Traditional (positivistic) scientific method focussed on hypothesis testing that involved seeking evidence to refute the hypothesis. Or to put it more simply this type of science begins with an idea about what might work, mindful that we can never be totally sure we are right as the next set of results might prove us wrong! This type of inductive reasoning created a frame or paradigm dictating the type of research question that could be asked and the ways in which scientists would test their ideas. Clinical trials draw upon this research tradition and the experimental paradigm.

There are however many aspects of knowledge and different ways of knowing that are important to integrated care and to explore these requires a paradigm shift that allows us to explore and make discoveries about experiences of living with dementia, dementia care and caring practices. Failure to choose an appropriate methodology could lead us to reject something of potential benefit to people with dementia or is supportive of family caring, simply because we used the wrong research lens to determine its contribution, or we tried to measure something that simply was not measurable.

Box 22.1 Reflective thought

How appropriate would it be to design a randomised controlled trial to demonstrate the efficacy of football reminiscence as discussed in Chapter 15? What other options might be considered?

If we reframe the way we think about dementia care within a bio-psychosocial integrated care model, positioned within rights-based approaches this will shape what and how we investigate. It will challenge ideas about people with dementia being research subjects moving us towards possibilities of research partnerships and collaborations. Initiatives such as The Dementia Engagement and Empowerment Project (DEEP) have been influential in harnessing the collective voice of people with dementia and involvement groups (Williamson 2012). Testimony to the success of this movement has been the increased involvement of people with dementia and family carers within service development and evaluation in the UK.

There are different knowledge bases and discourses that shape applied dementia research and health/care service research, and if you read examples of work across just three decades you will notice substantial changes in approaches to research which mirror the different ways that our views about dementia have emerged and changed over time with a current emphasis on partnerships in practice and involvement in research. The Evidence Based Practice movement that seeks to make explicit the evidence informing best clinical decisions has had to wrestle with unresolved tensions and continued debates about the nature of evidence and the practical challenges of equipping practitioners to access and apply the evidence where they work (Booth et al. 2011).

There are numerous calls for practitioners to provide dementia-friendly interventions and care environments. In the hospital environment this would be reflected, for example, in the ability of staff to organise work around the needs of people with dementia rather than being restricted to ward routine. The Handley et al. (2016) review concluded that staff training as a single strategy is insufficient to change practice and that the organisational culture needs to change to legitimise the practice changes required for best practices to become embedded. Handley et al. also recognised the lack of clarity on patient outcomes in research and this means that it can be difficult for staff from different disciplines to appreciate the benefits of dementia-friendly practices if they do not see this in terms of demonstrably beneficial outcomes. The Scottish Dementia Champions Programme, discussed in Chapter 13, is one of the few national initiatives that addresses this from a broad understanding of personal outcomes for people with dementia by equipping practitioners to be change agents promoting state of the art practices.

Which evidence matters?

The prevailing paradigm dictates which sources of evidence are deemed to have merit (Pearson et al. 2007). In health and social care this is about whose knowledge is most prized, is it that of the practitioner, the recipient of care, the family carer or research-based knowledge? In dementia care the presumed wisdom of the practitioner has been shown to be most useful when this is coupled with personal knowledge and partnerships with individuals and family. An example of the scope and range of knowledge that is required to deliver best practice in advanced dementia care is illustrated in the European Palliare Best Practice Statement (Holmerova et al. 2016). The six domains of practice-based knowledge detailed in the Palliare Best Practice Statement show the complexity of advanced dementia care and the breadth of evidence that is required to inform and shape these domains for practice. This begs the questions of which evidence matters and is required to inform such inter-professional learning frameworks. To answer this question it is helpful to return again to questions about the way we think about our practice, the practice models which shape our approach and the values and evidence bases which guide our decision making. We contend that the answer lies in a continuum of approaches whereby a diversity of evidence is required, but that the balance of the different forms of evidence and ways of knowing will vary with the questions we set out to answer. If we want to understand the experience of care, then we must foreground, respect and value the voice of the recipient of that care with an appreciation of practitioner perspectives. If we want to understand aspects of diagnosis we must focus on biomedical knowledge, mindful of the acceptability of possible evidence informed approaches to the individual who is seeking a diagnosis, the cost, risks, clinical usefulness and accuracy of the results.

If we embrace a person-centred approach to care it follows that evidence must include the voice of the person with dementia. However, in advanced dementia care there are many quiet voices that can be difficult to hear as discussed in Chapter 11.

> **Box 22.2 Discussion point**
>
> Think about a practice problem that you are interested in exploring. What types of evidence will assist you to gain understanding? How accessible are these different forms of evidence?

Designing research to advance practice

Research ideas are plentiful in practice and there has been growing interest in the development of what are often described as non-pharmacological interventions. Cognitive Stimulation Therapy (CST) is an example of a brief group programme intervention, design to help people with mild to moderate dementia. The key aims of CST are to improve cognitive functioning using techniques that exercise different cognitive skills. This is based on the principle of "use it or loose it". Clinical trials have shown a range of improvements including with language, executive functioning and quality of life with 14 sessions of CST (Spector et al. 2003, 2011). Maintenance CST, that is sessions continued over a longer time period, are helpful and particularly so when combined with medications (Orrell et al. 2014). Building upon the success of group-based CST, a recent development has been to test individualised CST administered by family carers in the family home, with mixed results (Orrell et al. 2017). This latest study should not lead us to reject individualised CST but to ask questions about the context in which it might work best including who delivers it and how its benefits might be amplified when used in combination with other approaches. An exciting advance might be to combine CST with a novel treatment of repetitive transcranial magnetic stimulation. This innovative non-invasive form of brain stimulation is also designed to improve cognition in Alzheimer's Disease through modulating neuro-plasticity which might in turn increase receptivity to cognitive training (Rabey and Dobronevsky 2016; Zhao et al. 2017). The possibilities of different combinations of non-pharmacological therapies offer promising new avenues for future applied research and for techniques we are yet to imagine as part of everyday practice. Once we have developed new approaches the next challenge is to get this new knowledge into practice.

Getting new knowledge into practice

The impact of practice-based research on experiences and outcomes of care is directly related to the use we make of this evidence within practice and services. Despite the rhetoric of evidence informed dementia care there remains a persistent gap between what we do and what we know from research would improve outcomes and care experiences for individuals and family. In a recent systematic scoping review of 88 studies addressing dementia research dissemination and implementation, Lourida et al. (2017) report that few studies involve people with dementia or family carers. They highlight gaps in evidence-based dissemination and implementation particularly within hospital and primary care settings. The review authors explain a plethora of implementation barriers and incomplete reporting of dissemination and argue that efforts to implement what is already known within dementia care is at best naïve and at worst recklessly wasteful. This situation they contrast to other areas of practice where more sophisticated approaches do seem to bridge the evidence practice gap. As we discuss earlier within this book the evidence base much underpinning dementia practice and caring interventions is of variable quality and an abundance of small studies is no substitute for a robust evidence base for practice. It also follows that if confidence in the underlying evidence is weak that this will understandably lead to cautious implementation efforts. The moral question that practitioners need to address is what type of evidence and how much of this evidence do they require before they implement that which appears to be helpful or desired given the current state of the art and science of dementia care.

Conclusion

Evidence based dementia practice is a complex undertaking due to the progressive nature of the underlying illness and the many ways that the dementia experience changes and challenges lives. The dementia experience is undoubtedly rooted in illnesses that damage the brain, the consequences of which manifest in an array of changing health and social care needs. Accordingly we need to build evidence that can negotiate this and inform interdisciplinary practice. We also need to create modern integrated dementia services that enable and support individuals to live the best life possible at all stages of this condition.

References

Booth, J., Tolson, D., Schofield, I. and Lawrence, M. (2011) "Applying Evidence to Practice." Chapter 2 in Tolson, D., Booth, J. and Schofield, I. (eds) *Evidence Informed Nursing with Older People*. Oxford, UK: Wiley-Blackwell.

Handley, M., Bunn, F. and Goodman, C. (2016) "Dementia friendly interventions to improve the care of people living with dementia admitted to hospitals: a realist review." *BMJ Open*, 7(7). Available from: http://dx.doi.org/10.1136/bmjopen-2016-015257.

Holmerova, I., Waugh, A., MacRae, R., Veprkova, R., Sandvide, A., Hanson, E., Jackson, G., Watchman, K. andTolson, D. (2016) *Dementia Palliare Best Practice Statement*. Paisley, Scotland: University of the West of Scotland.

Lourida, I., Abbott, R.A., Rogers, M., Lang, I.A., Stein, K., Kent, B. and Coon, J.T. (2017) "Dissemination and implementation research in dementia care: systematic scoping review and evidence map." *BMC Open Access*, 17: 147. doi:10.1186/s12877–12017–0528-y.

Nutley, S., Walter, I. and Davies, H.T.O. (2003) "From knowing to doing: a framework for understanding the evidence-into-practice agenda." *Evaluation*, 9: 125–148.

Orrell, M., Aguire, E., Spector, A., Hoare, Z., Woods, R.T., Streator, A., Donovan, H., Hoe, J. and Russell, I. (2014) "Maintenance Cognitive Stimulation Therapy (CST) for dementia: single-blind, multicentre, pragmatic randomized controlled trial." *British Journal of Psychiatry*, 204: 1–8.

Orrell, M., Yates, L., Leung, P., Kang, S., Hoare, Z., Whitaker, C., Burns, A., Knapp, M., Leroi, I., Moniz-Cook, E., Pearson, S., Simpson, S., Spector, A., Roberts, S., Russell, I., de Waal, H., Woods, R.T. and Orgeta, V. (2017) "The impact of individual Cognitive Stimulation Therapy (CST) on cognition, quality of life, care giver health and family relationships in dementia: a randomised controlled trial." *PLoS Medicine*, 14(3): e100226

Pearson, A., Wiechula, R., Court, A. and Lockwood, C. (2007) "A re-consideration of what constitutes 'evidence' in the healthcare professions." *Nursing Science Quarterly*, 20: 85–88.

Rabey, J.M. and Dobronevsky, E. (2016) "Repetitive transcranial magnetic stimulation (Rtms) combined with cognitive training is a safe effective modality for the treatment of Alzheimer's disease: clinical experience." *Journal of Neural Transmission (Vienna)*, 123(12): 1449–1455. doi:10.1007/s00702–00016–1606–1606

Spector, A., Thorgrimsen, L., Woods, B., Royan, S., Butterworth, M. and Orrell, M. (2003) "Efficacy of an evidence-based cognitive stimulation therapy programme for people with dementia: randomised controlled trial." *British Journal of Psychiatry*, 183: 248–254.

Spector, A., Gardener, C. and Orrell, M. (2011) "The impact of Cognitive Stimulation Therapy groups on people with dementia:views from participants, their carers and group facilitators." *Ageing and Mental Health*, 15(8): 945–950.

Williamson, T. (2012) *A stronger collective voice for people with dementia*. York: Joseph Rowntree Foundation.

Zhao, J., Li, Z., Zhang, J., Tan, M., Zhang, H., Geng, N., Li, M. and Shan, P. (2017) "Repetitive transcranial magnetic stimulation improves cognitive function of Alzheimer's disease patients." *Oncotaget*, 16(8): 200. doi:10.18632/octotarget.13060.

Index

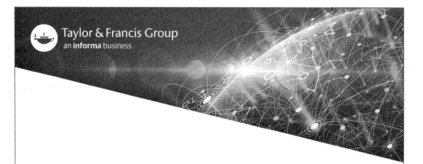

Printed and bound by CPI Group (UK) Ltd, Croydon, CR0 4YY

21/10/2024

01777040-0003